"Autometrics"

A complete manual on how to workout in your car!

Introduction

This title is bound to raise some eyebrows, and I would be surprised if it didn't.
How in the world can you workout in your car?!
If you are envisioning doing pushups across the bench seat of your pickup while driving on cruise control, you have the wrong idea, I assure you!

Another question might be why would you want to do that?!

I can answer both of the above questions very easily!
I for one have a very long and tedious commute to work every day, and I suspect I'm not alone in this.
I try to make my drive time at least somewhat productive by listening to informative talk radio, books on cd, how-to cds, and things like this, fairly often.
Sure, sometimes I just crank up the tunes and settle for a little entertainment; I'm not a TOTAL nerd!
However, I am always looking to make what would be boring, tedious "downtime" more productive and less mentally draining.

Table of Contents

Pure Isolation Flexing

KSHD Exercises

More "conventional" equipment usage in the car

Putting it all together

Instead of sitting around and doing nothing while you're driving, you can at least do a couple of things that can give you more energy and revitalize you," notes Canadian physiotherapist Maureen Hagan, who has just been named personal trainer of the year by IDEA, a group with 20,000 fitness and health professionals.

(This is a quote from an online fitness article found here): http://www.washingtonpost.com/wp-dyn/content/article/2006/08/14/AR2006081400879.html
I paraphrased a couple of other exercise ideas from this article in some of the pages below.

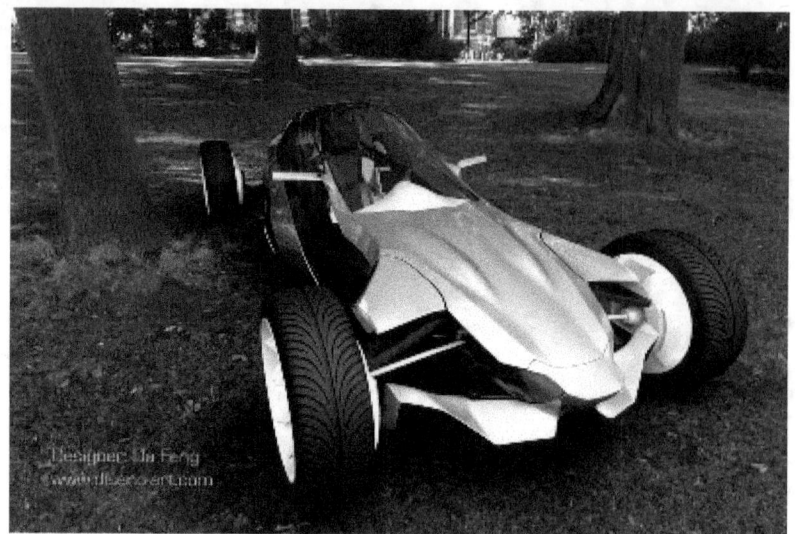

Workout in the GYMCAR shown above

Now, if you have the green and want to "go green", you can opt for this really cool "Gymcar" I found featured on the internet.

You can see the diagram below which shows how the interior design is made with working out while you charge the car's batteries (it's obviously a hybrid model) in mind.

What you're looking at above is the GYM Car concept designed by Coventry University design student Da Feng. As you might guess, its design incorporates exercise equipment that allows the driver to take his or her workout on the road.

The GYM Car itself is a single-seater with a lightweight, injection-molded, magnesium alloy chassis and carbon fiber bodywork.

The GYMCAR is powered by an electric motor with batteries that can be recharged by plugging it in or, and here's the interesting part, through the use of the onboard workout machinery.

 When the vehicle is parked, the driver can use any or all of the built-in equipment to generate electricity for the charge. There's a stepping machine and rowing machine available using the sliding seat, pedals and steering wheel. There's also a bench press or pull up simulator that uses the seat and an overhead handle.

The arm rests can even be used for curls thanks to their tensioned resistance. Pretty much any move you make inside the GYM Car will burn calories and generate electrons at the same time. Check out more renderings in the gallery below.

I found this "*car of the future*" at this website address:

http://www.autoblog.com/2008/12/12/gym-car-concept-gives-you-a-good-workout/

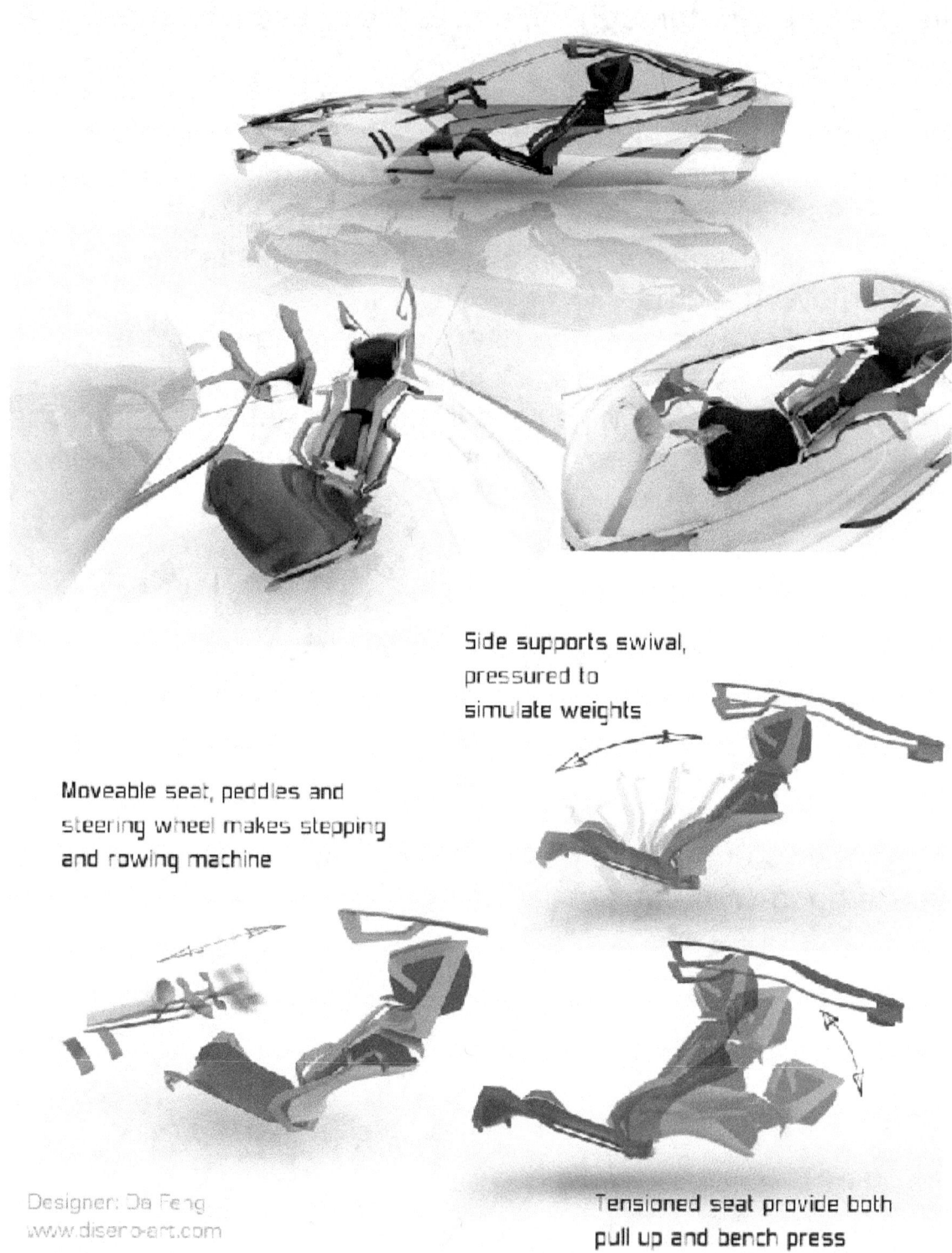

Side supports swival,
pressured to
simulate weights

Moveable seat, peddles and
steering wheel makes stepping
and rowing machine

Tensioned seat provide both
pull up and bench press

This was not quite what I had in mind when I started writing this book, but I found it while garnering info from online sources to add to my own ideas.
While this is a super cool concept, it is probably beyond the means of most of my target audience.
I know it's beyond mine!

For those of us who are trying to workout in our "Normal" vehicles, I've put this stuff together which I hope you will try.

I have been doing a lot of this stuff myself and am constantly trying to figure out more ways to try.
I hope you will **think outside the box** and come up with some additional exercises and ideas yourself.

☺

While I have a reasonably well set-up home gym, it is not always easy to get more than a couple of workouts a week in, what with everything else I have on my plate.
Again, I suspect I am not alone here.

One of the aspects of training and keeping all the joints in good working order, that I tend to neglect or slack off in, is the area of **flexibility or stretching.**
If something is going to be cut short from one of my workouts, this area is a likely victim, even though I know I should not neglect this.

It occurred to me that some form of stretching could be done **in the car,** while commuting, and especially when stuck in traffic and the car is not moving at all.

Of course, a full body, thorough stretching routine might be a bit tough to achieve in the car, but you can definitely get some stretching done, as I have learned.

Also, in my research for my recent book "**Forgotten Secrets of the Old Time Strongmen**", I came across some very interesting older routines which required no special equipment, and some of which required very little space in which to perform the exercises.

Later, I started to frequent forums on bodyweight exercises, and some new terms came up and aroused my curiosity.

Really, the new terms were just "catch phrases", used mostly by folks selling exercise programs based on long pre-existing routines.

The terms were **DVR (Dynamic Virtual Resistance), Iso-tension, Dynamic Tension, Virtual self resistance, KSHD**, and some others.

"**Dynamic Tension**" was the term used by **Charles Atlas** for his isometric and self resistance courses which are still being sold to this day.

KSHD stands for Kin Shi Hai Do, which is an ancient martial art form which basically translates to lifting weights without the weights, or "**virtually lifting**".

Probably all of these concepts had their roots in ancient martial arts traditions that have been revamped, rehashed and re-hyped in more modern times.

What all of these methods have in common is that **they can be done sans equipment,** though some can be aided or enhanced in some cases by the use of equipment.

While I read the older routines that consisted of these types of methods with considerable interest, I was at least a little skeptical of their effectiveness, and therefore did not immediately incorporate them into my normal training regimen at first.

When I started reading proponents of these methods posts on forums, blogs, e-books and in other such places, I started to consider these methods with a little more interest than previously.
In truth, there are quite a few purveyors of such methods on the net and elsewhere these days that seem to have quite the loyal following.

I decided to try some of the suggested exercises, and found them not at all unpleasant, if perhaps not quite as taxing or effective as one of my typical powerlifting workouts.
I have incorporated some type of bodyweight exercises in my routine for a long time, and have always thought they had some value. I have told folks starting a routine, who maybe could neither afford to join a gym nor buy expensive equipment, *that one could develop a decent strength training routine using bodyweight exercises alone*.
I still think this is true.

In Arnold's "*Education of a Bodybuilder*", which I read with relish as a younger man, he suggested a number of bodyweight style exercises as a precursor to heavy weight training for novice trainees, but I think one could even build on such a program and *create a more advanced program without the use of weights, if one so desired*.

Another methodology I became familiar with earlier in my powerlifting "career" was *PNF stretching*.

PNF stands for **Proprioreceptive Neuromuscular Facilitation**.

These are big words, and the science behind them gets a little complicated, but the practice of PNF stretching is not all that complicated, in reality.

It involves an **assisted stretch**, preferably with another person, but an inanimate object such as a wall (read car seat, head rest, etc for the purposes of this book), can be used also.

In this type of stretching, one performs a mild stretch, and then **exerts some force as in an isometric contraction**, but not exerting max effort. The **force can counter the resistance of a partner or that of the afore-mentioned inanimate object.**

The first position is held for a count of 5-7 seconds or so. Next, one would relax very briefly, before going into a slightly deeper stretch and duplicating the same method as in the first position.

Several rounds of this are done, until the maximum "comfortable" position is reached, and then one would move on to another position.

Dr. Fred Hatfield, the first powerlifter to squat over 1000 pounds in an official power meet, was a big proponent of this method of stretching, and it was in one of his books that I first read about this concept.

Some of the PNF style stretches lend themselves well to our purposes in this book, and will be delved into in more detail later.

Static stretching is another type of stretching, and is probably more familiar to most folks and highly recommended by fitness professionals everywhere.

This requires **simply holding a stretched position for a longer period of time.**
Again, **some of these types of stretches can be done in the car,** so we will discus several of these in this book as well.

Even if you did no other types of exercises in your car other than stretching, you will have better spent some of your otherwise "wasted" commute time in something **more useful, healthy and productive.**
That is a great place to start, I think.
I intend to show you lots of other exercises beyond simply stretching that will be a little more challenging, however.

Of course, there are a few downsides to this type of routine.
For one thing, the person driving the car next to yours might just think you are an escapee from the nearest sanitarium.
I don't concern myself too much with this one; the heck with them if they can't take a joke.

Another item is getting overly distracted in concentrating upon the exercise and not your driving.
There are ways around this, most obvious of which is to only do the exercises during longer traffic stops.
You can set your **cruise control** when driving on the highway at a relatively fixed speed, which will free your feet up from having to be on the pedals constantly.

Another idea is to start out with the less complicated and strenuous movements until you get used to doing them while driving, and then gradually work in the more strenuous and complex moves over time.

The one form of exercise that requires no real movement would probably be a good place to start, as there is minimal distraction involved, both for yourself and the nosy onlooker driving alongside you.

Of course, if that nosy onlooker happens to be a State trooper, you may want to take a short breather until he passes you!

Can you do exercises with little or no movement?? YES!!

I know it sounds a little strange at first, but I think you will be won over once you really put your mind to it and give it a valid attempt.

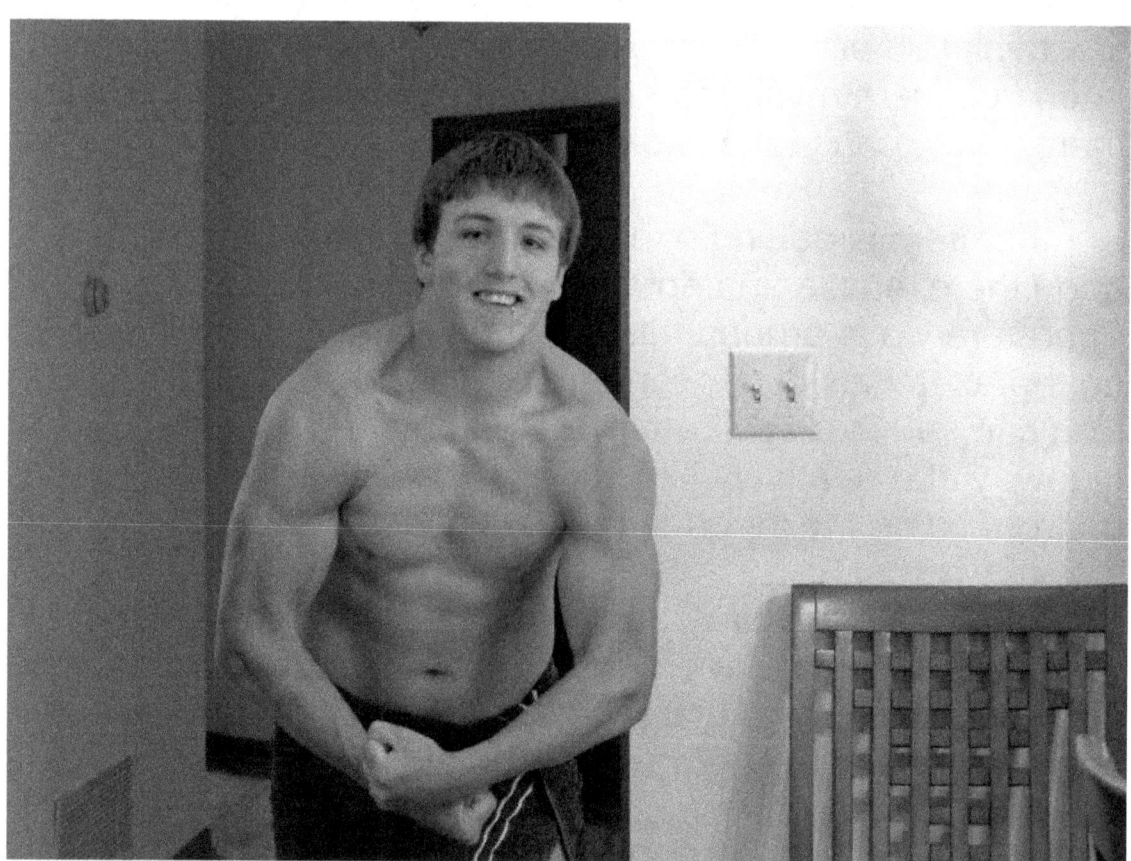

My Stepson Kevin striking a classic pose

Flexing/Contracting

Have you ever seen a bodybuilder flexing in the mirror, going from one pose to the next?
This is written off by the masses as narcissism, but the bodybuilder is not simply admiring himself or herself when doing this. (At least, not always)
Besides practicing for an on-stage posing routine, designed to display one's physique to the best possible advantage, this posing/flexing actually hardens the muscles, makes them more vascular (veins visible and not covered by fat layer) appearing, and can even provide additional growth.

Just flexing the muscles can be fairly taxing, depending on the number of positions, the length of time they are held, and the amount of effort put into the flexing.
It is not too difficult to flex hard enough and long enough to actually induce cramping in the targeted muscle, as some of you may already be aware.

While you can find various catchy sounding exercise routines that incorporate muscle flexing, it is nothing new, and I am certainly not claiming to be its inventor.
This is without any doubt the most practical and simplest form of exercise you can do while driving.
There are also isometric exercises and **KIN SHI HAI DO** exercises that can also fit very well into the traveling fitness routine road show.

I think it is best to learn as many different types of movements as you can, so you have a large "*tool box*" from which to pick.

I think we can even learn a few tricks from *Yoga and Pilates* manuals, as well as *Qi gong*, *tae chi* and similar methods. In fact, I ran into a DVD being advertised on the internet for something called "carlates", about doing a limited Pilates routine in the car.

We can probably incorporate some more *traditional exercise modes,* but *with certain adaptations* so that they can be done in the car.

I am not going to suggest that you will become Mr. Olympia by training in your car or that you will lose 20 pounds of fat and gain 10 pounds of muscle over the next 6 weeks but *I do think you can make your commute more fun and productive by doing these exercises.*
You will arrive at your destination feeling *more refreshed and less stressed out,* I am sure.

You will gain a little strength and flexibility and become more "*in tune*" with your body and its muscles.
It costs nothing, will make you feel better, and you will be wondering how the time went so quickly.
I have been practicing some of these exercises on my commute lately, and find them to be a nice addition to my "traditional" workouts.

If this is the only exercise you can manage to squeeze into your busy schedule, *you will certainly be better off than had you continued to do nothing.*

I am going to suggest some additional types of exercise that you can sneak in during your work day or at home, which will only enhance your conditioning, but these are optional, of course.
If you do already exercise at a gym or at home,
but find it tough to get all the workout time in that you would prefer, these methods will provide a valuable adjunct to your other training without being a time drain.

If you have little or no background in weight training or other strength training exercises, it may be difficult getting the hang of some of the movements from the onset, but I think most will get the feel for them with a little patience and persistence.

One of the basic concepts that must be learned is simply **flexing a particular muscle or muscle group in an isolated fashion (by itself)**.
I think most of us, especially men, can remember using or hearing the phrase "**make a muscle**" generally referring to flexing the biceps and posing in such away as to display the flexed muscle.
You would just concentrate on contracting or flexing the biceps as hard as you could, without also contracting the triceps, forearms, deltoids, or other muscles at the same time.

Flexing or contracting multiple muscle groups at the same time is not a taboo subject, but **it is better to learn to control each muscle individually for best results in what we are trying to accomplish in this program.**
So if you can think about the way you "made a muscle" with your biceps and apply that to any muscle in your body, you are well on your way.

Another concept that comes into play in the more advanced lessons is that of "**antagonistic**" muscles.
These are muscles that **stabilize or "brake"** against a contracting muscle with an "**opposing**" force.
The triceps would apply the opposing force against the biceps, in one situation; the hamstrings group (back of leg) would oppose the quadriceps group (front of leg).

When I speak of "**isolating**" a muscle, I am talking about a muscle group, as opposed to an individual muscle.
The biceps is a muscle "group" consisting of 2 heads, for example, and the triceps is composed of 3 heads.
The front of the leg is composed mainly of the quadriceps muscle group, which as you might guess, contains 4 heads.

The upper back muscles are the **latisimus dorsi, the trapezius, rhomboids,** and some other smaller muscles.
To try and isolate one head of the triceps or the biceps and flex just that head would be difficult, at best, though traditional weight training exercises often are said to hit one part of a muscle group more strongly than others, largely because of the positioning and technique used.

For our purposes, **I will be expecting you to flex/contract the entire muscle group** when I write: flex the frontal leg muscles or quadriceps, as an example.

You must have some knowledge of **human anatomy** and muscular structure in order to know what muscles I am speaking of and where they are located, as well as their primary function.

We do not need to learn the Latin names of every single muscle, but just a very basic understanding will be helpful.

In the following diagrams borrowed from an old muscle control course written by **Ed Jubinville** and made available on the *Sandow plus website*, you will see both frontal and rear view diagrams of the main muscles of the body.

Study these and become familiar with the terms and you will be better prepared to embark on our exercise routine.

This is not an all encompassing diagram set, and does not go into super detail, but it will serve our purposes very well.

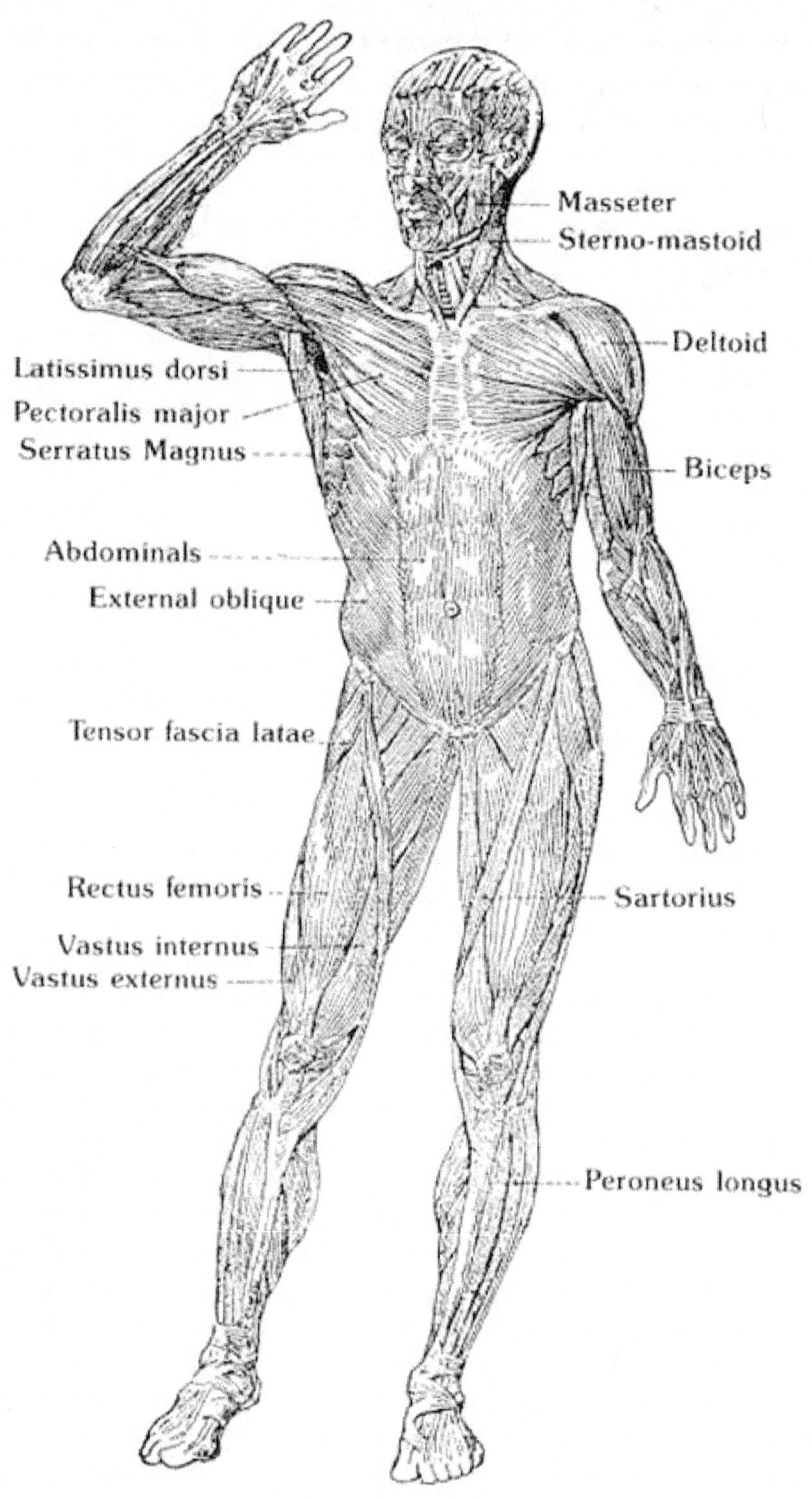

Masseter

Sterno-mastoid

Deltoid

Latissimus dorsi

Pectoralis major

Serratus Magnus

Biceps

Abdominals

External oblique

Tensor fascia latae

Rectus femoris

Sartorius

Vastus internus

Vastus externus

Peroneus longus

106

18

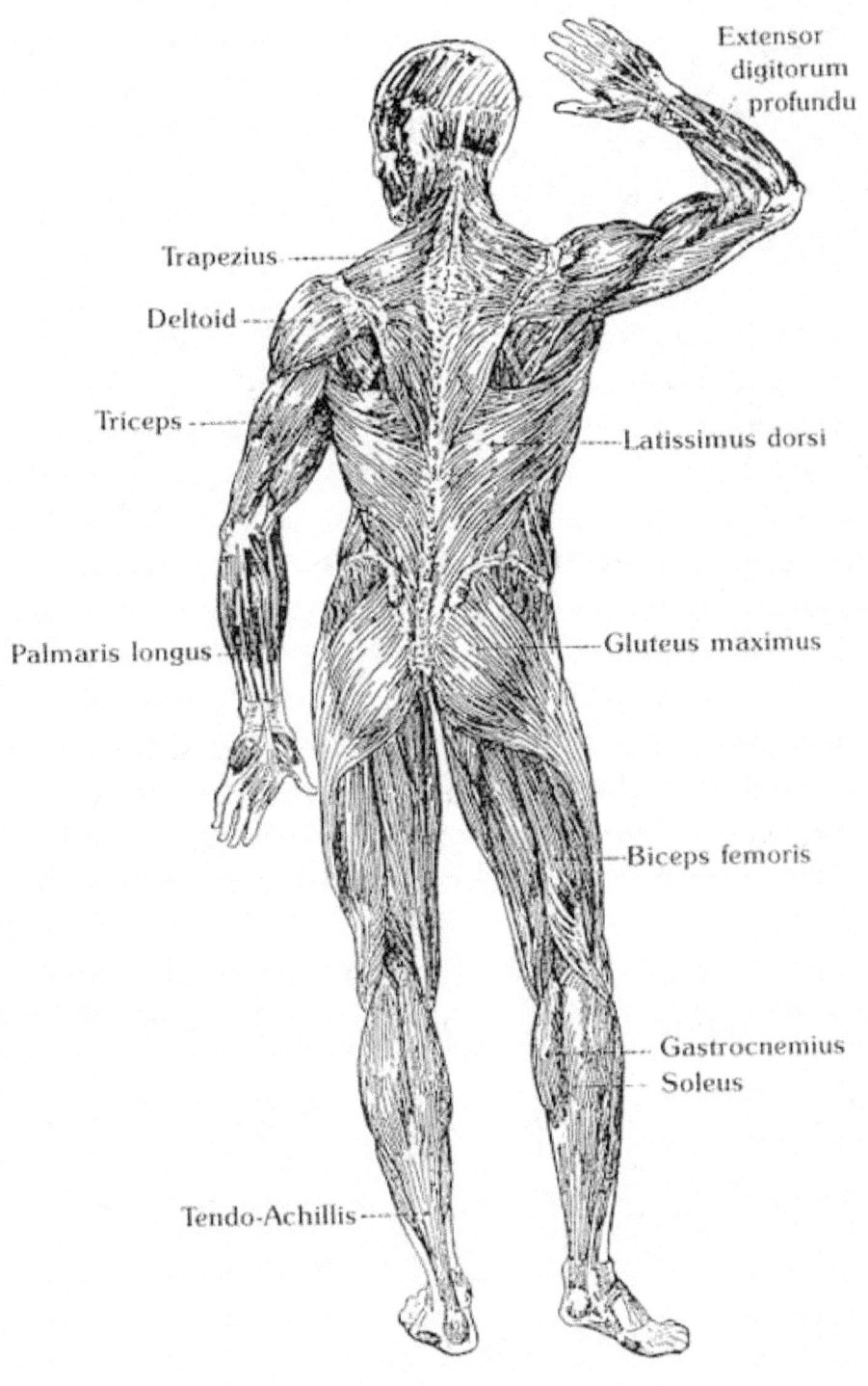

Extensor
digitorum
profundu

Trapezius

Deltoid

Triceps

Latissimus dorsi

Palmaris longus

Gluteus maximus

Biceps femoris

Gastrocnemius

Soleus

Tendo-Achillis

107

19

Some terms you may not be familiar with if you are new to exercise are "**sets and reps**".

A set is one short period of exercise, consisting of a number of repetitions, or "**reps**".

In weight training, one might perform 3 sets of 8 repetitions in a given exercise, for example, before moving on to another exercise.

In the pure flexing exercises, **we will typically hold a flexed or contracted position for a set time period**. Counting seconds in the old "one Mississippi, two Mississippi", etc. style has always been a useful tool to me, but use whatever counting method you like. Just be consistent with it.

You will **fully relax the involved muscle (s) in between repetitions, just momentarily, before each consecutive repetition.**

So, when I suggest doing 10 repetitions of a bicep flex/hold, you will be expected to flex/hold for a given time period (perhaps 7 seconds), then relax for a second or two, and then follow with similar reps/rest until all ten are completed in this fashion.

We may do **multiple sets** for each body part, or simply go from one part to the next in more of a "**circuit training**" style.

We could also follow a **flexing type of movement** with a **stretching type of movement** for the same body part.

I have always been an experimenter, and I like to try different schemes to see which feels best.

We must keep in mind that **muscles need time to rest and relax after being exercised, in order to grow.**

It is not a good idea, then, to train the same muscles 2 days in a row, at least in a strength training format.

Stretching trained muscles is acceptable, as long as a little restraint is used.

This is another area in which **antagonistic muscle groups** comes into play.
I like to think in terms of "**pushing**" or "**pulling**" exercises, but I will admit this is a bit of an over-simplification, as not every muscle fits exactly into one category or the other.

If I train "**push**" muscles on a given day, then I will train "**pull**" muscles on the following workout day.

In other words, I might train the legs, upper back, biceps and forearms one day, followed by shoulders, triceps and pectorals on the next workout day.

The neck muscles can fit into either of these 2 groups, but I tend to think of them being tied to the pectorals more than the upper back, though they really have attachments to both. Abdominals can fit into any workout, but it is usually suggested to not train them on consecutive days, as they need time to recover as any muscle does.
Calves are done on the same day as the rest of the legs, usually.

If you do other training, such as weight training at the gym or at home, do not follow an upper body, "**push**" style workout with weights or using bodyweight, with another "**push**" style car workout the next time you train, unless these training days are several days apart.

Try to keep your training **balanced** between pushing and pulling, or upper and lower body parts, regardless of what training format you are using.

If you feel you have a **weak area**, less developed than others, it is fine to put a little more emphasis on that area, but do not fall into the trap of training a favorite or stronger part to the exclusion of the rest of the body.

This leads to one over developed area and other under developed areas. **This can cause injuries, muscle imbalances, poor symmetry, and a less attractive and less functional physique.**

You probably have seen guys that look like cartoon characters because of this syndrome (think POPEYE, with massive forearms and little else that would be impressive)

Deep Breathing

There is **another thing that is easily accomplished while driving and yet provides great benefits to our health and wellness.**

The concept of **Deep Breathing** has been around for thousands of years, and this is yet another idea that was touted over and over again in old-school programs from the past.

Yogis and martial artists have been practicing some form of this for a very long time, and I think it's a good thing to add into any fitness program.

I can just imagine the skeptics among you that are now thinking; "oh, great, now this genius is going to teach us to breath"!

"Somehow, I have managed to stay alive for x number of years without having had this training, so I think maybe I can survive without it a little bit longer"!

Well, you are absolutely right, you can certainly **survive** breathing just as you have been since birth.

The funny thing is that **you are probably not breathing just as you were right after you were born.**

Babies practice deep breathing instinctively, right after that first smack in the rear given soon after leaving the shelter of the womb.

Watch a baby's respiration sometime if you have the opportunity.

You will notice **the belly rising on each incoming breath, and falling somewhat on each exhalation.**

Somehow, as we grow older, many if not most of us "re-learn" to breathe in an improper fashion that is less than optimal.

We can survive just fine breathing this way, yes, but we can do better if we re-learn **the original way**.

Most of us practice shallower breathing than we are capable of, and this prevents us from having the best of health.

Nasal breathing is always preferred to mouth breathing, and should be practiced whenever possible.

The only thing that should or might prevent it is having a stuffed up nose.

With a bad sinus condition, an upper respiratory condition or allergies, there may be some difficulty, obviously, with this type of breathing, but try the best you can to breathe through the nose **whenever possible**.

The nose contains "**filters**" which air passes through during respiration, that take impurities out of the air before it can reach our lungs.

Of course, the impurities or foreign matter then become trapped in our mucous membranes, but are easily dislodged by blowing the nose, or sneezing (the body's way of forcing out foreign matter).

Different trainers have slightly different takes on exactly how to perform deep breathing, but to put it into its simplest terms,
I would say just to try and take in as much air with every breath as you possibly can.
Think of the incoming air filling the lower abdomen, then the diaphragm, and finally completely filling the lungs on each and every breath.
This should not be "staged" into 3 or more separate breathing components, but become *one continuous, flowing inhalation of breath, followed by an exhalation that kind of works from the top down, and ends with the lungs being completely devoid of air.*
At this point, the lungs and body are "*primed*" for the next inhalation of life giving oxygen.

This is a *great thing to practice while driving, and especially in between "sets" of our other types of exercises*.
If you have ever been hypnotized, you may recall that in the initial stages, you are required to relax by *breathing very slowly, deeply and rhythmically.*
Deep breathing techniques can be a *great aid to relaxation* and associated reduction of stress, so I urge you to give it a try.
If you practice it often enough, your *normal breathing patterns will greatly improve, and you may even be able to slow down your heart rate, which is one of the often touted benefits of "cardio" training.*

Well trained runners or other practitioners of longer duration types of exercise typically have **slower resting heart rates**, which is a good thing.

Would it not be great to get some of that type of benefit without having to run for miles on a regular basis?

You may want to read more about deep breathing in a yoga manual or elsewhere.

There have been books written specifically on the topic, and I have just begun to scratch the surface of the topic here.

Well now, at this point we have discussed a few of the types of exercise that can be done while driving and/or while sitting in traffic.

We have mentioned **stretching, isolation flexing, and deep breathing** and discussed each briefly.

KSHD

I also mentioned something called "**KSHD**". This stands for **Kin Shi Hai Do.** To put it simply, this refers to the practice of performing weight training style movements without the weights, using "**virtual resistance**", supplied by one's own **antagonistic muscles.**

Various trainers have described this type of training in various ways, but you basically use "**internal resistance**" while **imagining pushing a heavy object or weight, or pulling down on ropes, pulling your own weight up to a chin up bar**, or something similar to these concepts.

It sounds kind of weird at first, yes, and I was just as skeptical as you probably are before I actually gave this a try.

Try to put your skepticism aside and give this a valid try, and I think once you start getting the hang of it, you will embrace it.

There are obviously limits to the type and number of these types of exercises that can be performed in the car, especially while actually driving, but there are at least a few that we will find suitable, I think.

If you learn a little bit of anatomy and think "**outside the box**" just a bit, you might be surprised what you can come up with on your own.

Getting Started

Reach Stretching

Stretching **comes naturally** to humans as well as animals. Have you ever watched a big cat at the zoo, or even your house cat at home simply reaching his front paws out as far as they can go? How about the classic back arch that is a Halloween favorite?

Consider some of the crazy stretched positions a cat or dog gets into while bathing itself.

Maybe some of these are not even intentional, but they do get the job done, none the less.

When you first wake up in the morning, you probably do a *yawning stretch*, simply reaching your arms and legs out as far as you can.

I mention these things simply to point out that **stretching does not have to be complicated or difficult.**
Just reaching an arm or leg out in any direction, as far as possible and holding the position for several seconds or more is an acceptable form of stretching.
When driving in your car, you can reach one arm at a time forward, backward, upward, or sideways.

Stretching the legs is tough to do this way, unless traffic is stopped, or you are able to take advantage of your cruise control setting, as you must use your right foot to constantly engage the pedals.
However, **during traffic stops or when using cruise control, you can stretch your legs quite a bit by using toe pointing or positioning of the ankles.**

Heel Raise

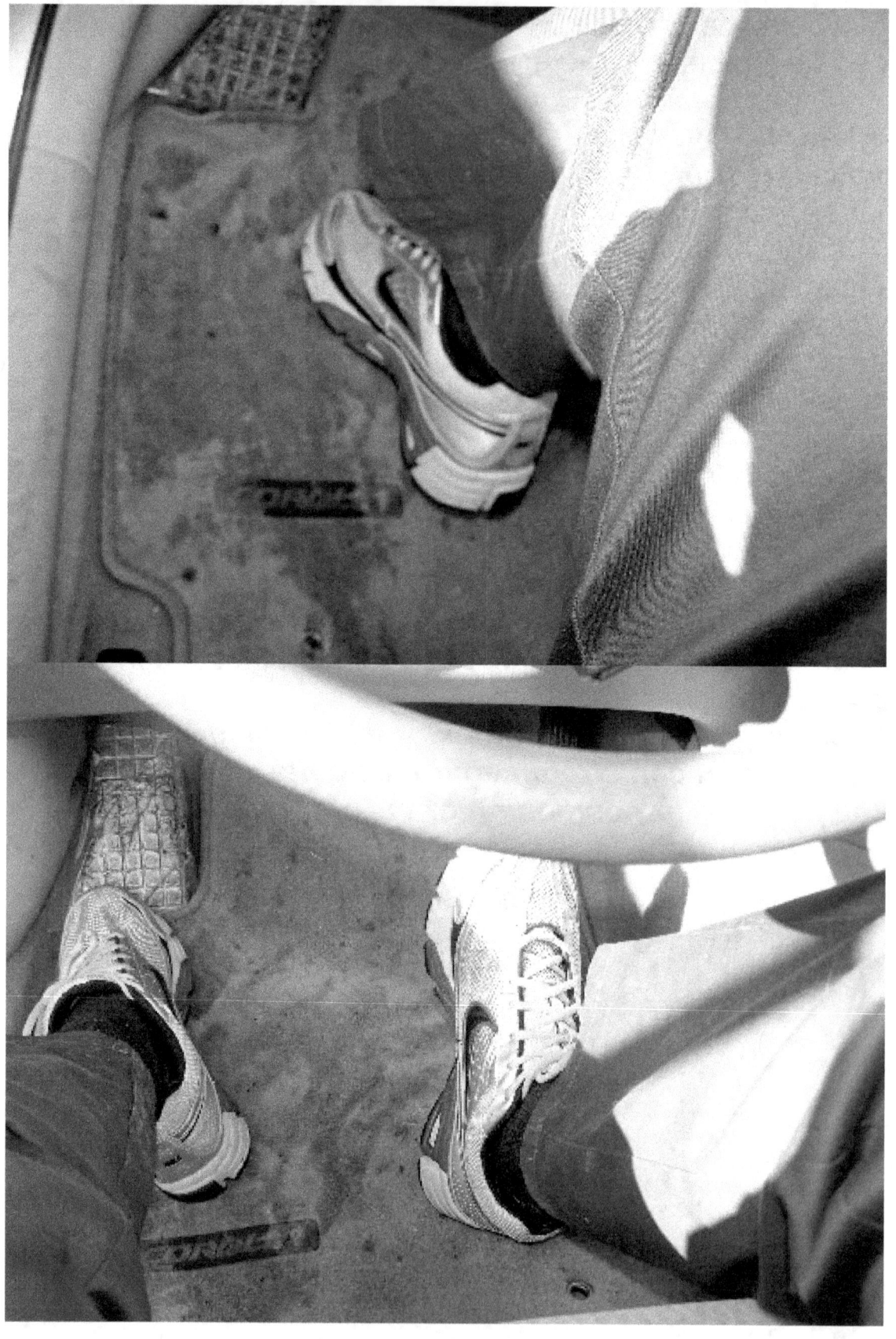

Stretching the Soleus, pointing toes backward

You can stretch your calves and soleus by **flexing your ankle forwards, while at the same time curling you toes downward**, hold that position for a short time, then **reverse the ankle and toe flexion so that you are trying to point your toes back towards your body.**

You can also **turn the feet as far as possible to either the left or right positions, again, as far to that position as is comfortable,** and hold the position briefly.
You will even feel these moves in your upper leg muscles.
You can also do **"twisting"** style stretches for the arms, by concentrating on various wrist flexion positions.

The **neck muscles** can be stretched in a similar fashion, by **"reaching"** your head back, forward, and to either side briefly as far as you can comfortably do so.

You can easily stretch the entire upper back and shoulder girdle area by **"shrugging"** your shoulders up as high as you can reach them, hold that position for a short time; then bring your shoulders back as far as is comfortable.
Try to **"squeeze"** your shoulder blades towards each other as you bring them back.
Now, reverse this and bring your shoulders forward and hold that stretched position again.
You can do a **"reverse shrug"** trying to pull both shoulders down towards the floor, and hold that position as well.

You can even "*roll*" the shoulders in a continuous forward, upward, backward, and then downward fashion while trying to reach the most stretched position in the sequence, or switch the sequence up in any way you see fit.

All of the above are forms of "**Static**" stretching, not requiring either **ballistic movements** or resistance applied against the stretch.

Assisted stretches can also be done in the car, and they are best performed during traffic stoppages, but are possible to do while the car is moving by using one side at a time. An example of this is "**hugging yourself**", in which you simply try to reach each hand as far around to the back of the opposite shoulder as possible. (from the front)

(There is an illustration of this a few pages forward)
You can stretch the shoulder by reaching as far as possible, or you can grab the opposite shoulder with the "reaching" hand and stretch or flex/contract the triceps muscle against the resistance of the held shoulder.
You will begin to see that stretching positions and isometric flexing/tensing positions can often, if not always, be interchanged.

Another good shoulder stretch that one can perform in the "**assisted**" style if both hands are free is done by reaching back behind the head with one arm, and **trying to touch as far down the middle of the upper back as possible**.

Another dimension can be added by also trying to "**push**" the elbow backward as far as possible simultaneously.
If the car is not moving and the hands are both free, you can "assist" the stretching arm by **pushing down on it with the opposite hand.**

Again, we can turn this into an isometric exercise simply by *flexing/contracting* the upper arm muscles *against the resistance of the opposing hand, and holding that contracted position for some time.*

Now we are starting to go into *another type of stretching*, beyond the "*reaching*" stretches we began with.

☼

Some PNF Stretches

As we already discussed, this type requires *pushing against a resistance during the stretch.*
Obviously, you will not be performing the assisted style of PNF stretching while driving, but rather *using parts of your car's interior structure or your own body for resistance*.

Again, it is hard to do some of these while the car is in motion, unless they are done with one arm at a time.

Using the headrest

You **can stretch the shoulders, triceps and pectoral muscles by using your headrest to push or pull against.** Reach back with either arm (or both, as shown in next photo) with its elbow pointing forward, and grab the back of your headrest.

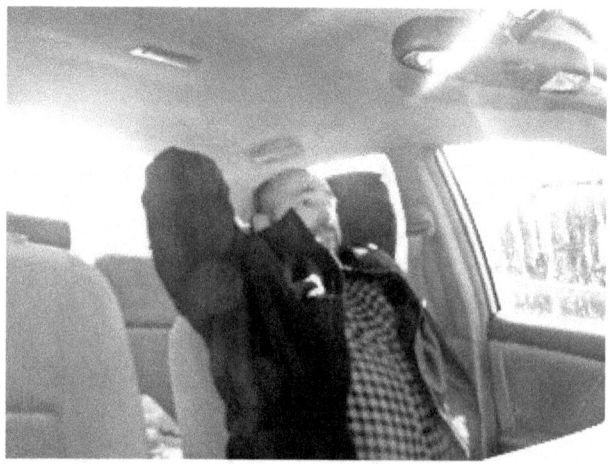

Reach back to just a **mildly stretched position at first**, and then hold firmly on the headrest while exerting some force against the headrest with the triceps muscle.
Hold that position for 5-7 seconds, and then relax momentarily.

Now reach back a little farther and grab the headrest firmly again and again follow by exerting some force against the headrest and holding for 5-7 seconds.
If possible, try one more, even deeper stretch to finish up. Follow with the opposite arm for the same sequence.

Next, you can do the same type of movement, but with the elbow facing out to the side this time.

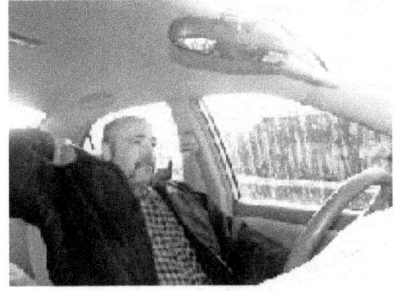

(Depending on what you are driving, this may not be practical, as there may not be enough room on **the left side**.)

Do it in this fashion for 2 or 3 stretched positions again, and then go to the opposite side and repeat.

One more move you can use the headrest for is to grab it by reaching back behind you, again with elbow out to side, but this time trying to stretch the elbow towards the rear.

Again, this may be tough in some smaller vehicles on the left side.

Using the roof

You can *use the roof as resistance to stretch the shoulders*.

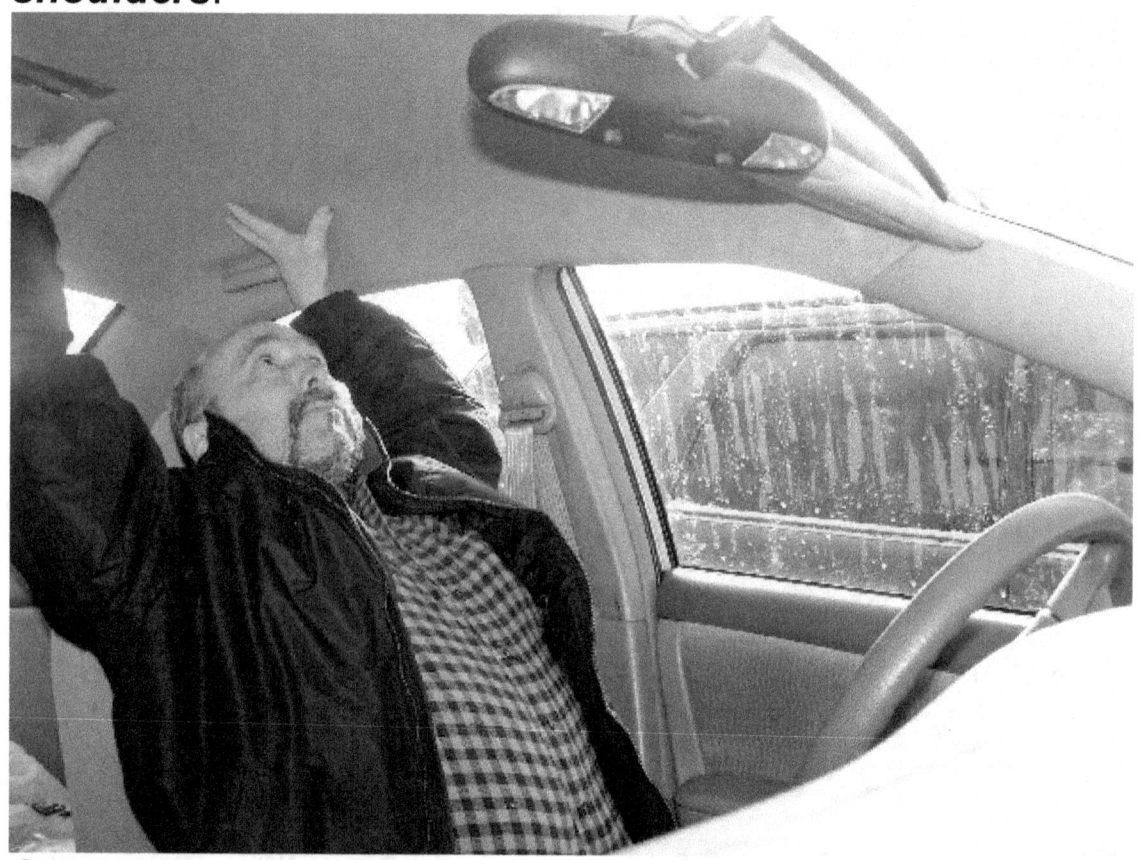

Stretching shoulders

Reach one hand up and back (or both during stops), putting open hand on roof.

Go for a mild stretch on the first position, and exert some force against the roof, hold for 5-7 seconds.

Rest for a couple of seconds, and then go for a slightly deeper stretch position, and again exert some force and hold for 5-7 seconds.

Repeat if possible, then switch arms and do same sequence for that side.

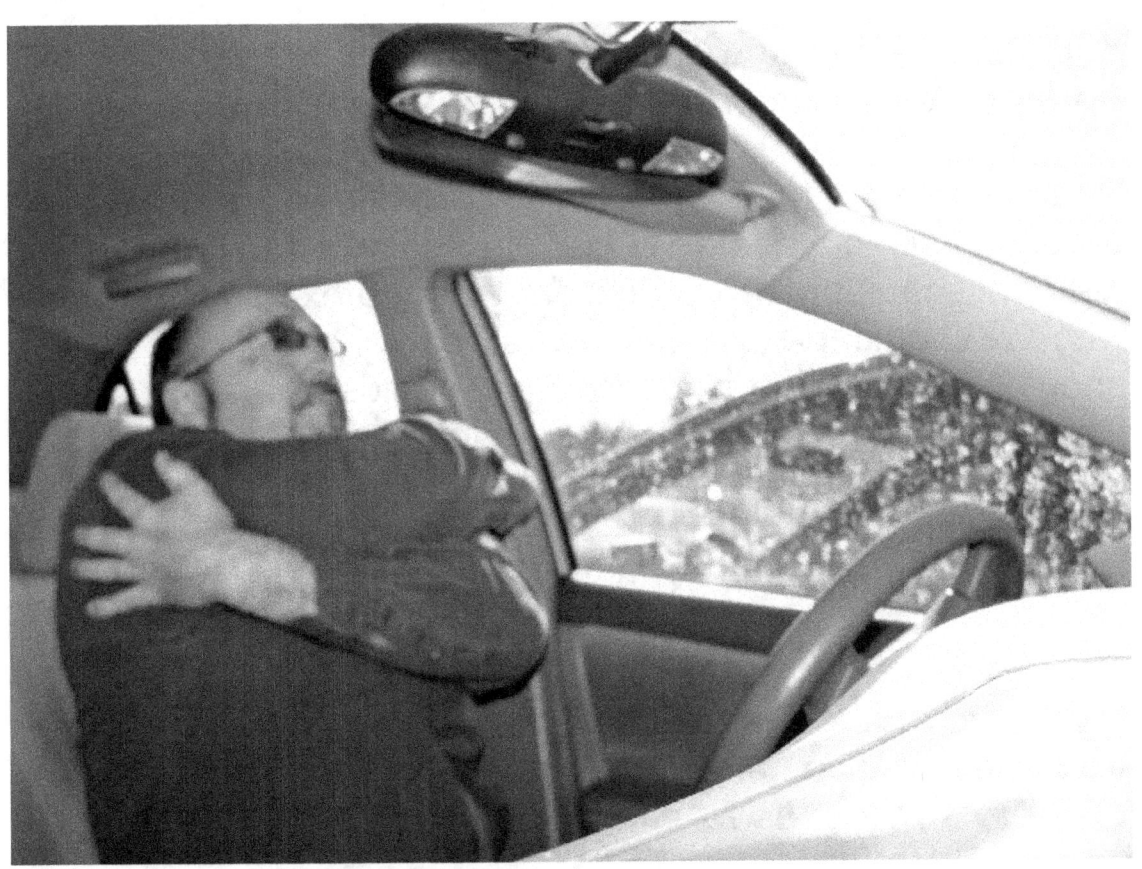

Reaching around right to left

Using your body

You can *use one body part to resist against another, both in PNF stretching and in isometric workouts.*

Reach your right hand around the front of your body and grab the back of your left shoulder. Reach to the point where the right shoulder feels a mild stretch, and exert some force with the shoulder against the resistance of your opposite shoulder. Hold the position for 5-7 seconds.
Rest for a second or two, and then try for a deeper stretch position and repeat until deepest comfortable position has been reached and held.
As usual, repeat same sequence on opposite side.

If you are stuck in traffic and the car is not moving, you can use one hand to resist against the other in order to stretch the forearms and biceps muscles.

To *stretch the forearm*, hold out one arm straight out and down in such a way that you can grab your wrist with the opposite hand.
Before grabbing the wrist, though, put a slight twist in the wrist of the stretched arm, in either direction.
Now grab the wrist with opposite hand and exert some force against the "*holding hand*" using the forearm muscles.

As we did before, hold this mildly stretched position for 5-7 seconds before relaxing briefly and following with a slightly deeper *twist/stretch.*

See Following picture illustration

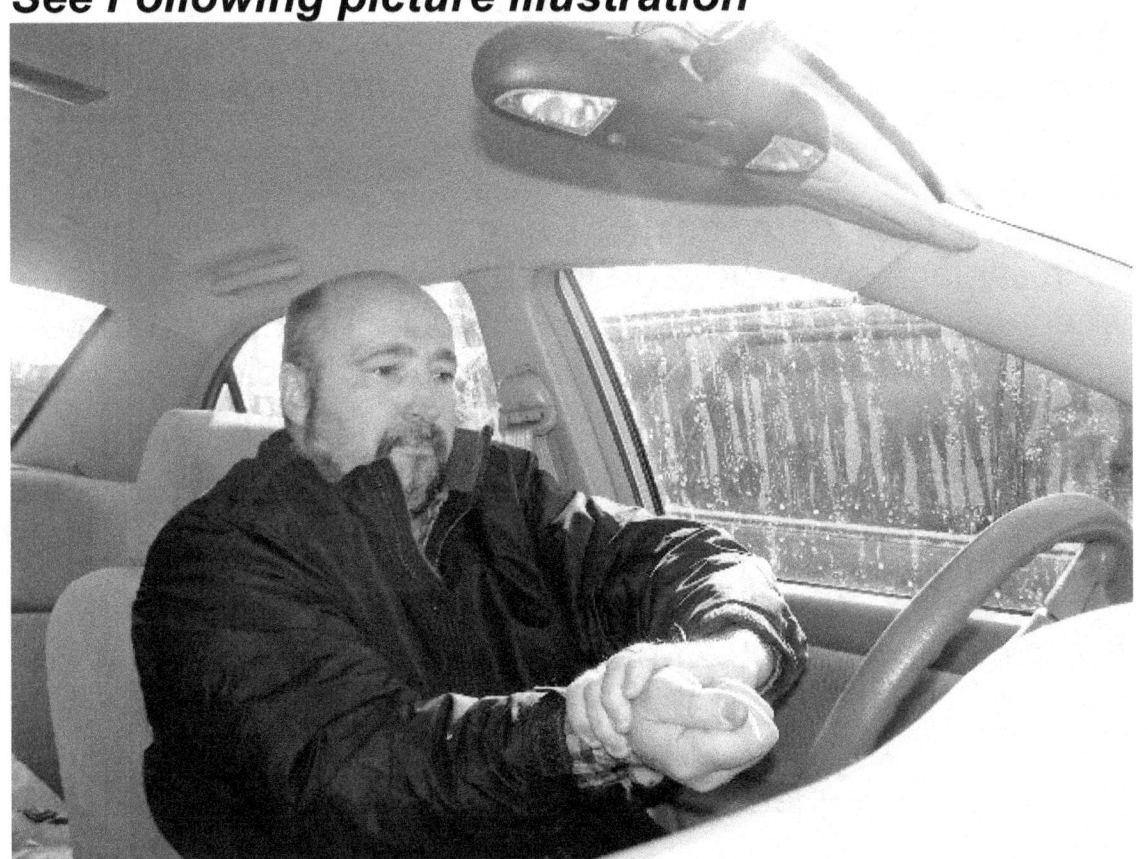

Hold the new position again for 5-7 count, and repeat until max stretch position has been reached and held.
Repeat with opposite hand, and then you can go back to starting arm and start twisting/stretching in opposite direction.
You can repeat the entire sequence with both arms twisting in this direction to complete the forearm stretching.

Of course, you may not be stuck motionless for long enough to go through this whole sequence.

If you suspect a short stoppage, Switch back and forth between opposite arms before going through entire sequence.

You don't want one arm thoroughly stretched and the opposite one neglected because of the timing.
When this happens, just try to start with the lesser worked arm/hand at the next opportunity.

To stretch the biceps, hold one arm straight out and down in a similar fashion as the last stretch started with, but this time when you grab the wrist with the opposite hand, exert force upward against the holding arm/hand with the biceps power, and go through the hold, rest method as previously described.

To **develop a deeper stretch, keep the hand of the arm that is being stretched open, and push down on the fingers of that hand with other hand to a new stretch position**.

Continue the sequence as in the above movements, for each side.

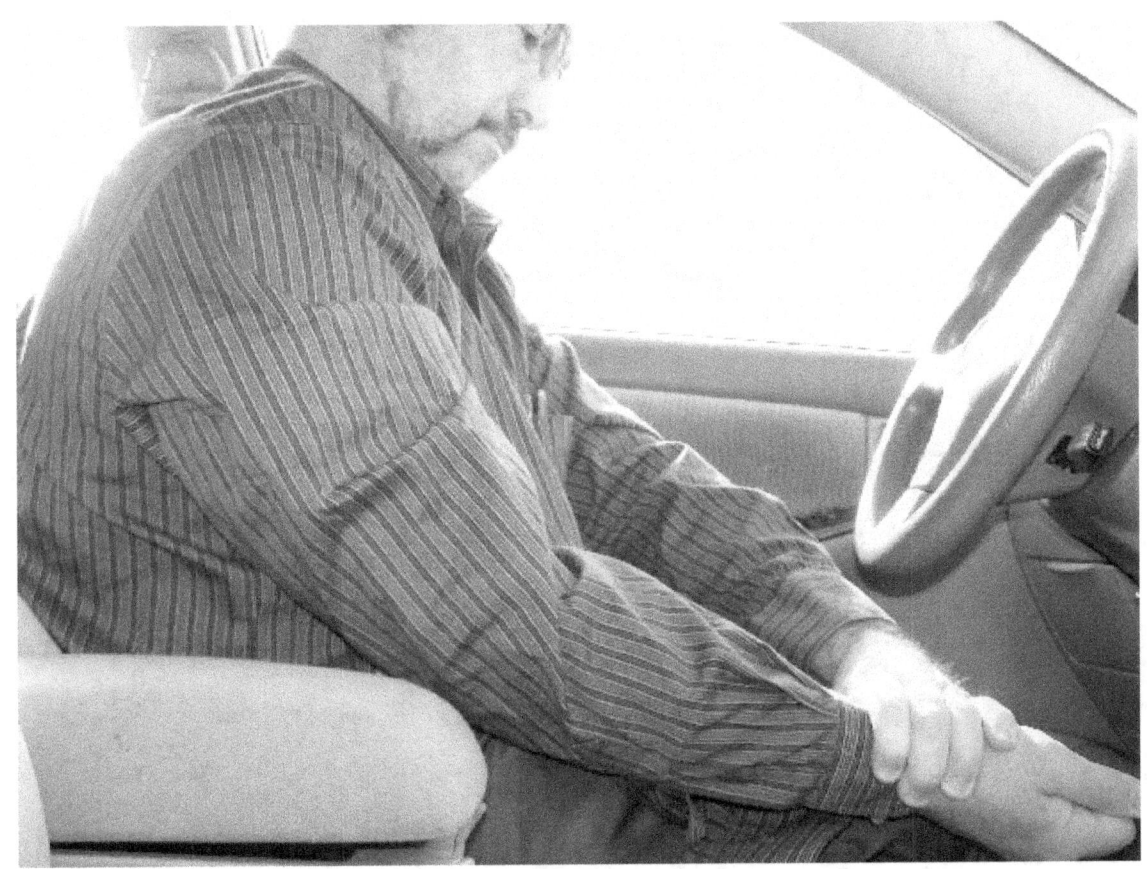

You can stretch the **triceps muscles** using a similar method also.

To stretch the triceps this way, *start by placing your right hand in front of you as if you were going to put your hand on your heart for the pledge of allegiance.*

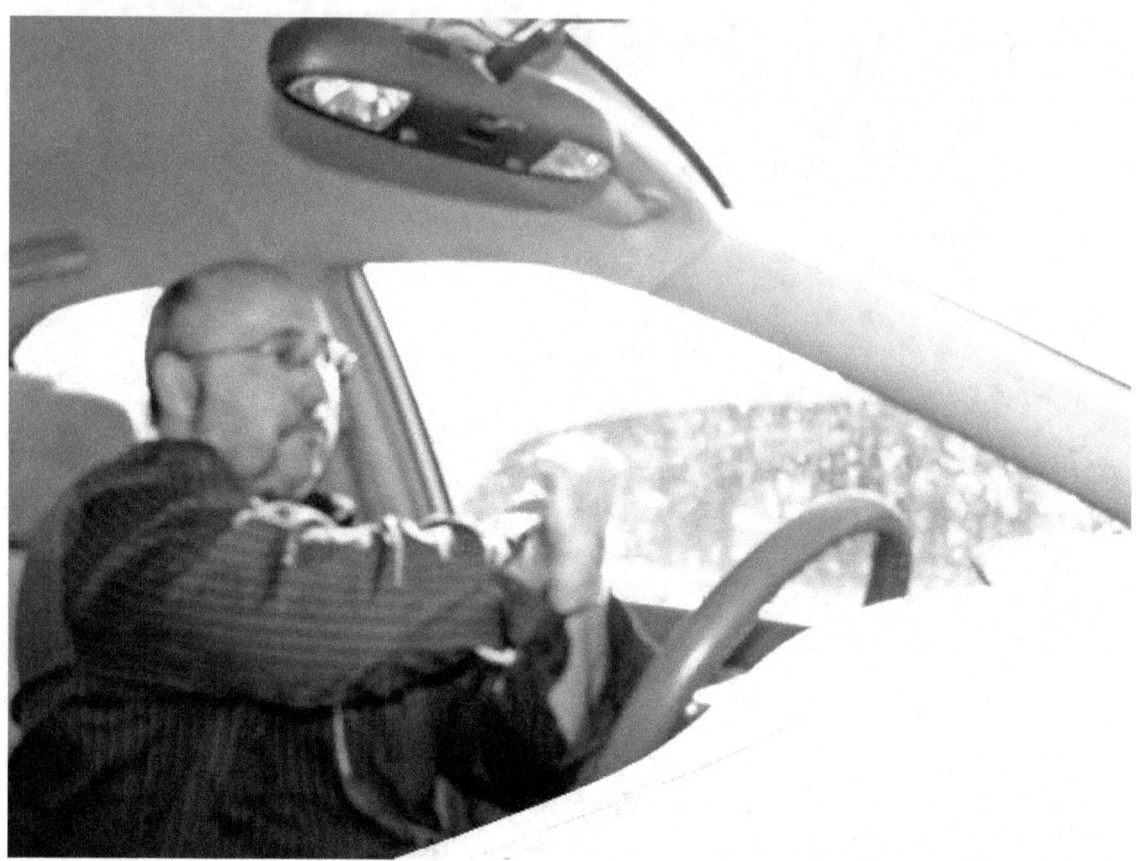

Now place your left hand straight up so that its wrist is directly in front of your right hand/wrist.
Keep the left arm rigid while pushing against its resistance with the Triceps muscles of the right arm, and hold the position as we did before on other movements. The closer you keep your left hand to the front of your body, the more the triceps will be stretched.
Start with the left hand out a bit so as to create only a mildly stretched position, and work it closer over the next couple of incremental steps.

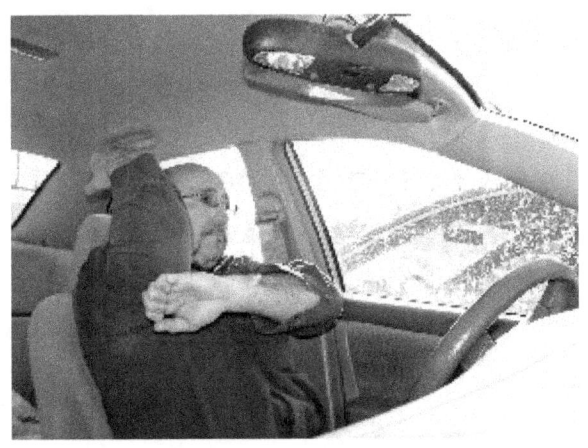

Another way to stretch the Triceps is to use the opposite hand to provide resistance, and start at the position shown, continuing to move the active arm higher with each position (Shown above)

Leg/hip stretches

When traffic is stopped or you are using cruise control on a long lonely road with no foreseeable interruptions, you can try this one:

Twist your right knee so that your right foot comes up towards your left leg.

Assist the right leg with your left hand, to a point where the foot is sitting either on the front of your seat, or better yet, on top of your left leg. Just holding that position in a "*static*" stretch may be all you can comfortably handle (if you can indeed get that far), but **you can intensify the stretch by pushing down against the right knee/upper leg area with your free hand.**

The harder you push down, the deeper the stretch will be that you can reach.

You can simply hold each new position for a count, or you can push against the hand that is pushing down the leg, using the hip and leg muscles.

Pushing down on leg for deeper stretch

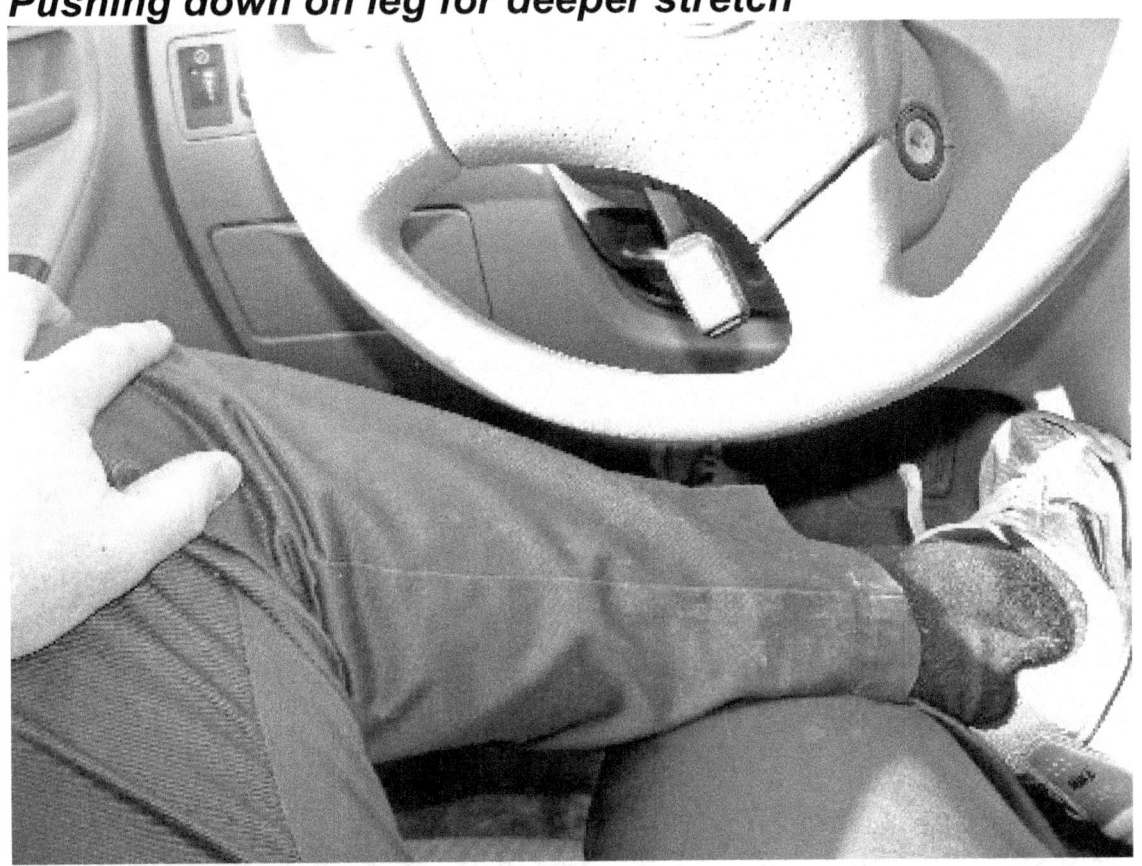

So, this can be done as a **static stretch, a PNF stretch, or an isometric contraction, or any combination thereof.** This will be true of many of the movements described.

Of course, you want to hit both legs this way, so simply reverse the directions to hit the other side.

Another leg movement is done by starting out in a similar fashion, but "**hooking**" the right foot behind the left leg and then "**pushing**" against the left leg's resistance with the muscles of the right lower leg.

The **closer the left leg is to your body, the deeper the stretch applied to the muscles**.
Again, start out with the left leg out somewhat so that the initial stretch is mild.
Repeat movement on other side.
This is **another movement that can be done as a static stretch, a PNF stretch, or an isometric contraction.**

Special Exercises
Posture Check

You can perform a posture check to prevent the ***driver's slump.***

In the car, sit up straight, trying to "***grow an inch***" taller by bringing your shoulders back. Lift your head so that your upper spine is erect and in more of a straight line. Retract your chin so that your ears are directly in line with your shoulders. Hold for 30 seconds while breathing in and out. Do a set of five to 10 reps.

Pelvic Floor Lift

Work your "*pelvic floor*". With age, added pounds and inactivity, the pelvic floor muscles grow limp. That increases the risk of both urinary and fecal incontinence and can compromise sexual function. Do "*Kegel*" exercises throughout the day to counteract the above issues.

Without using your derriere, draw up your pelvic muscles "*from the ground floor to first floor*," Hagan says, "*while also drawing in your belly button. They work best together.*"

(The above quotes were borrowed from an internet article by Dr. Hagan, who was quoted back at the beginning of the book.)

Shoulder Roll

Roll your shoulders up and then back while holding the steering wheel. *Gently pull your shoulder blades down and back toward your tailbone and your back pockets.*

This helps loosen shoulder and upper and middle back muscles, which tighten during stress.

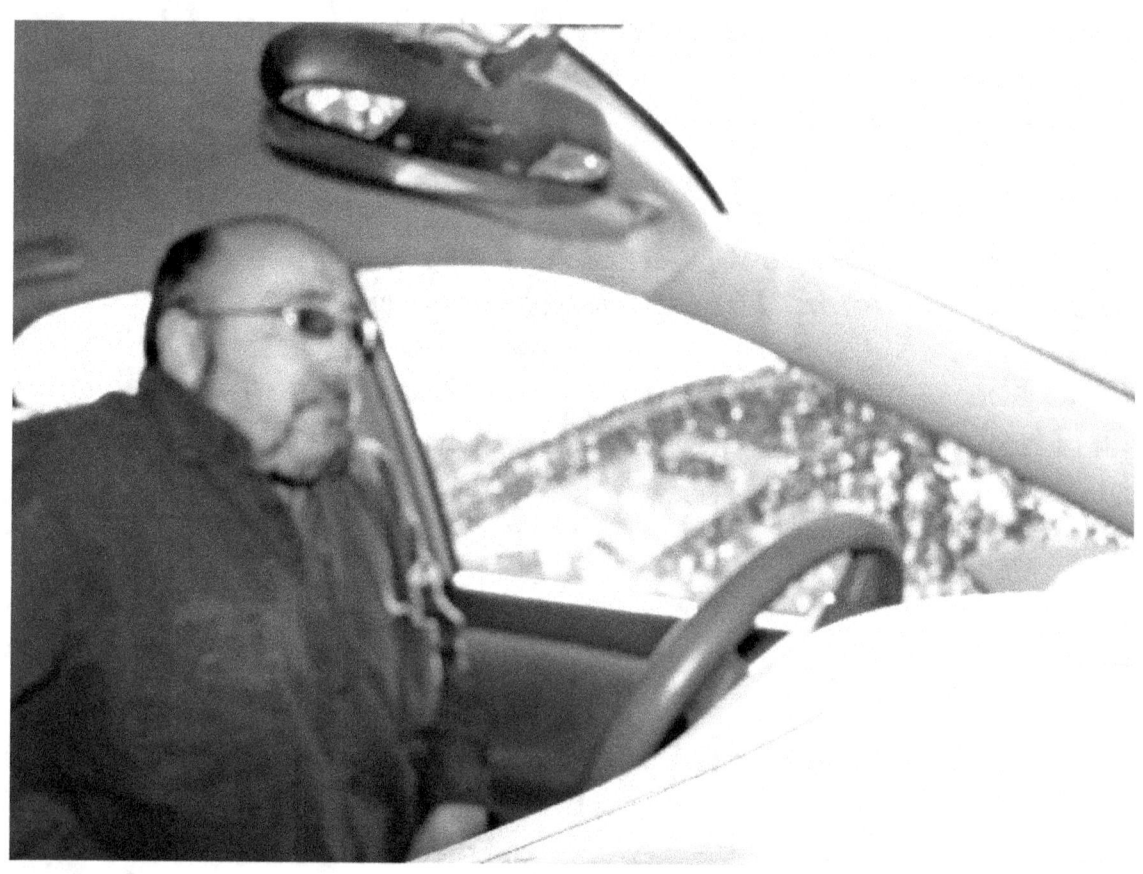

Shrugging/Rolling the shoulders

Isometrics

Using the steering wheel

You can **use your steering wheel for resistance in some isometric contractions.**

First, put your hands at the 9 and 3 positions (remember driver's ed?)

Push forward against the steering wheel and hold for 5-7 count.

Change your hand positions and **experiment with flexing different individual muscles (pecs, shoulders, biceps, forearms) or combinations of these muscles as you do this to get a number of different "feels".**

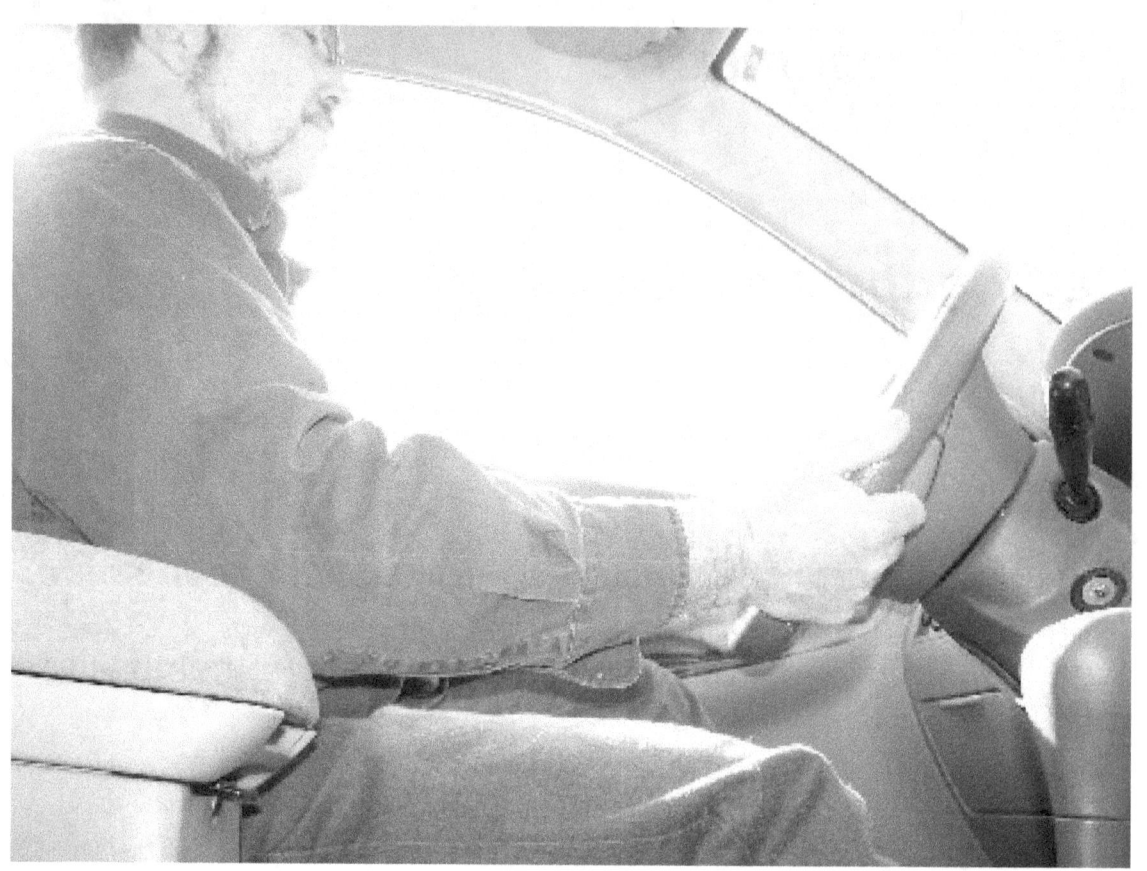

Gripping the wheel tightly

Grip the wheel

Clench as tightly as possible, concentrating on the hands, wrists and forearms, and then release.

At the same time, try to relax your shoulders. You can hold the grip for a count, or simply keep clenching and relaxing in a rhythmic pattern for some length of time.

You can also opt to push up against the wheel while flexing your Biceps.

Using a pillow

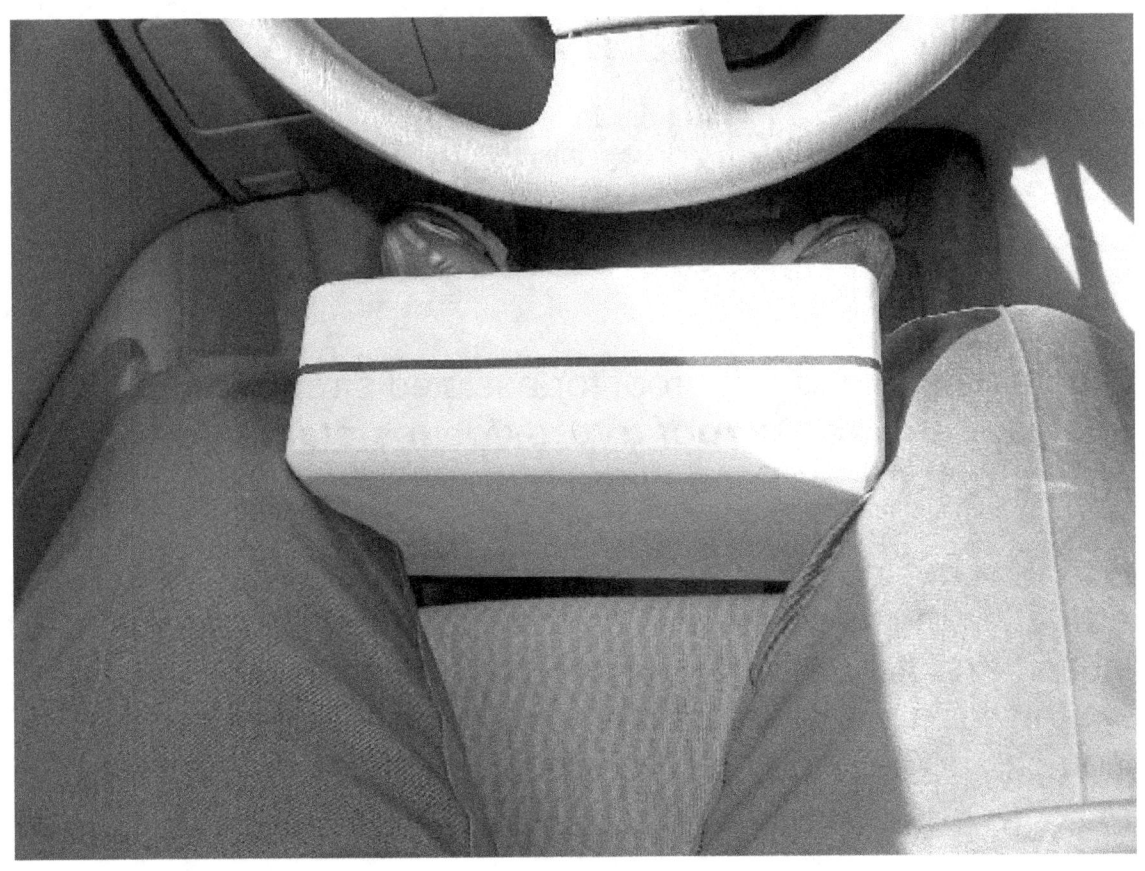

Strengthen your inner thighs.
Place a small pillow between your feet. Try to lift the item off the ground and squeeze your legs together at the same time. You can also **place the pillow or other soft object between your knees and squeeze**.
You can use the "***Squeeze/release***" continuously method for repetitions, or hold the contracted position for a count as in some of the previous movements.

Using the Roof

We discussed using the roof for assisted stretching already, and you can **use the roof to provide resistance for isometric contractions also.**

Simply reaching up and placing your hand (do this with 1 arm at a time while driving) on the roof and push against it, while flexing/contracting the shoulder muscles.
Do this for a 5-7 count as in the other isometrics we did.
You can do several "sets" for each side if you like before moving on.

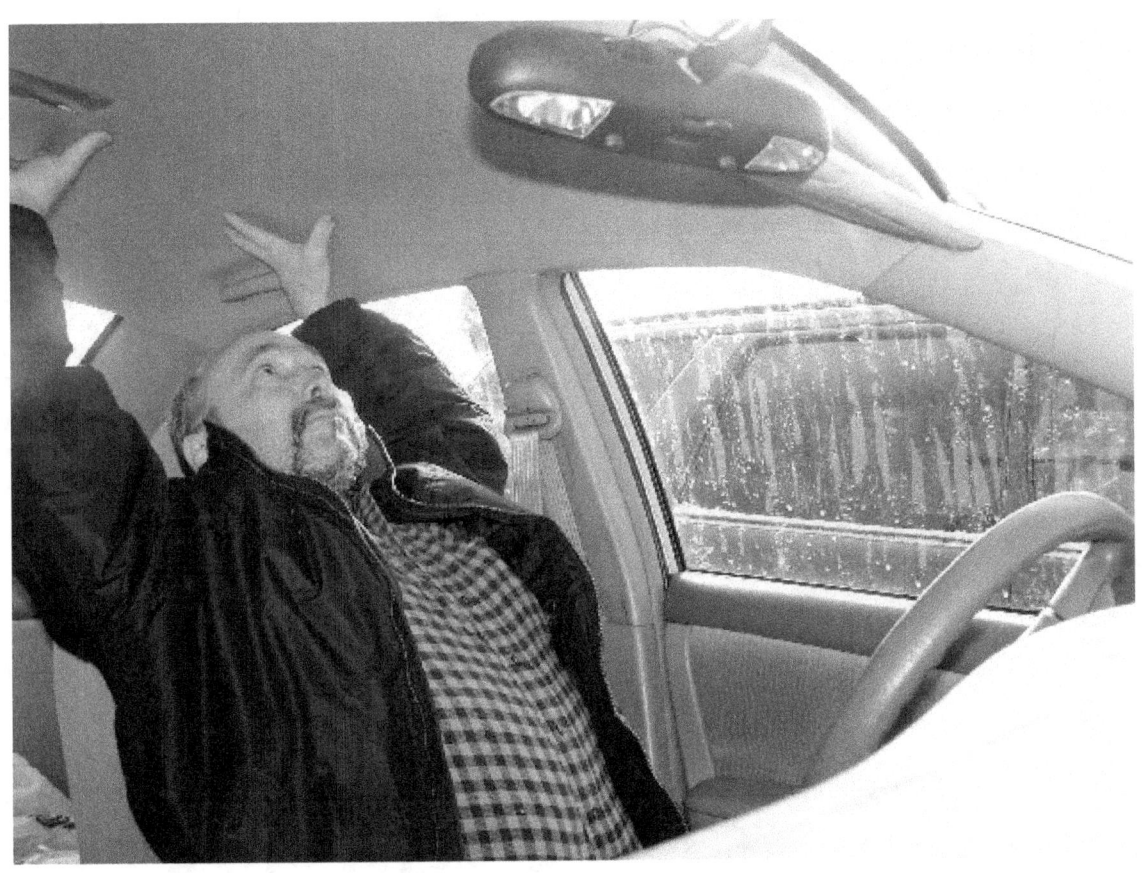

You can stretch and or do isometric contractions against the roof

If you want to feel more **pectoral muscle action**, you can **reach back at the same time as you reach up**, as **this puts some stretch and exertion on the upper chest.**

Flex the upper chest while also flexing the shoulder for this variation.

Using the dash/console area

Pushing right leg against right side of console

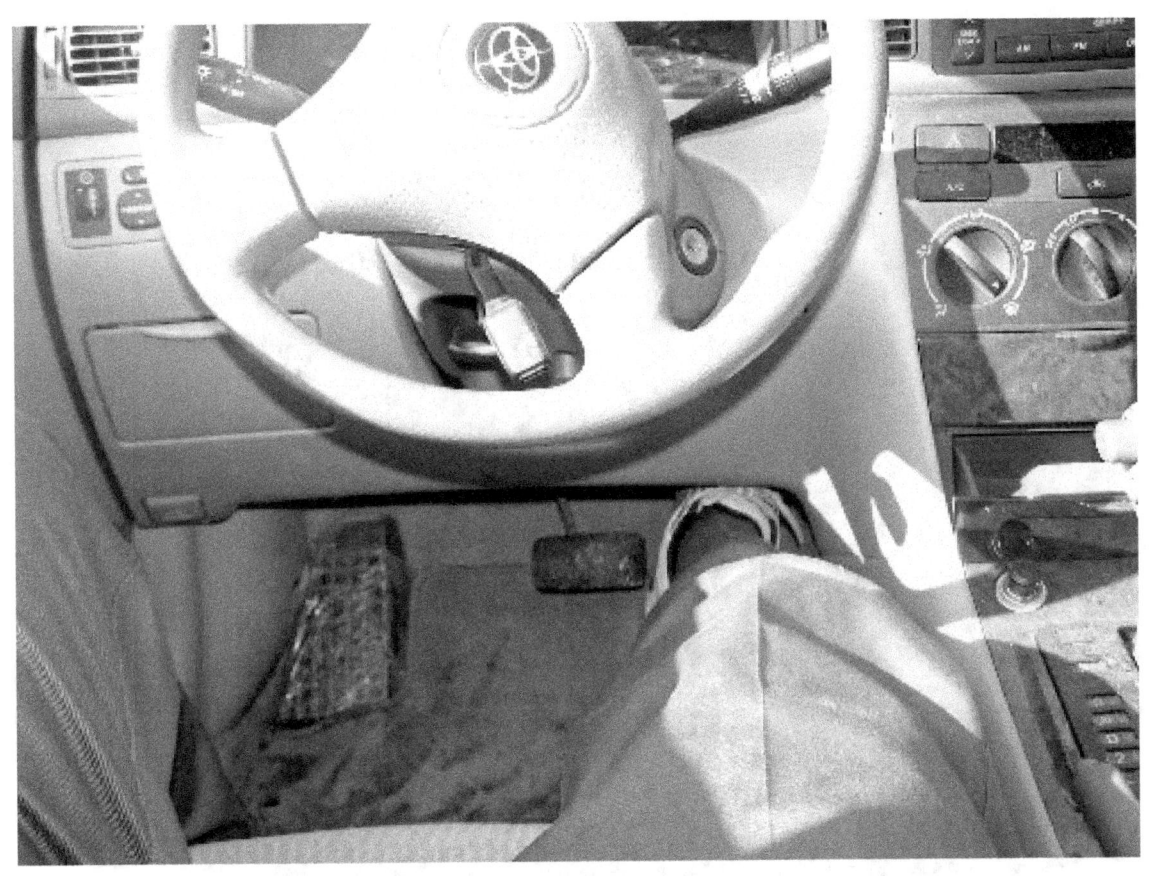

Pushing both legs upward against console/dash

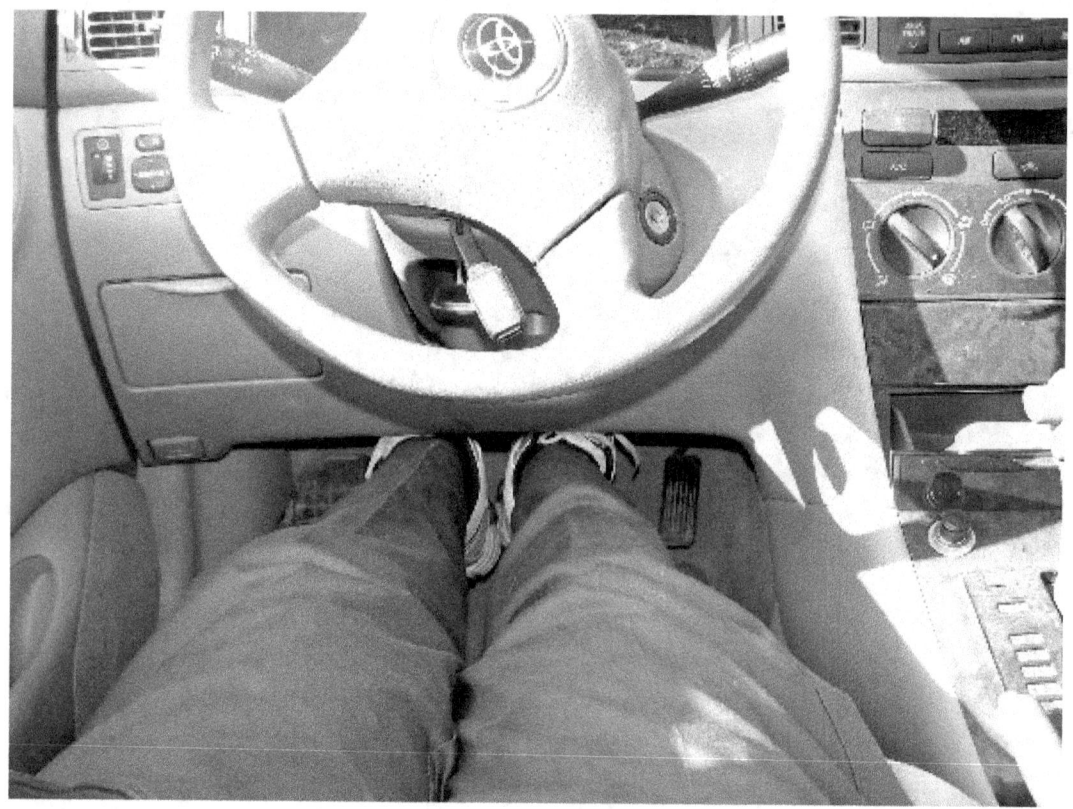

Pushing left leg against left side of console

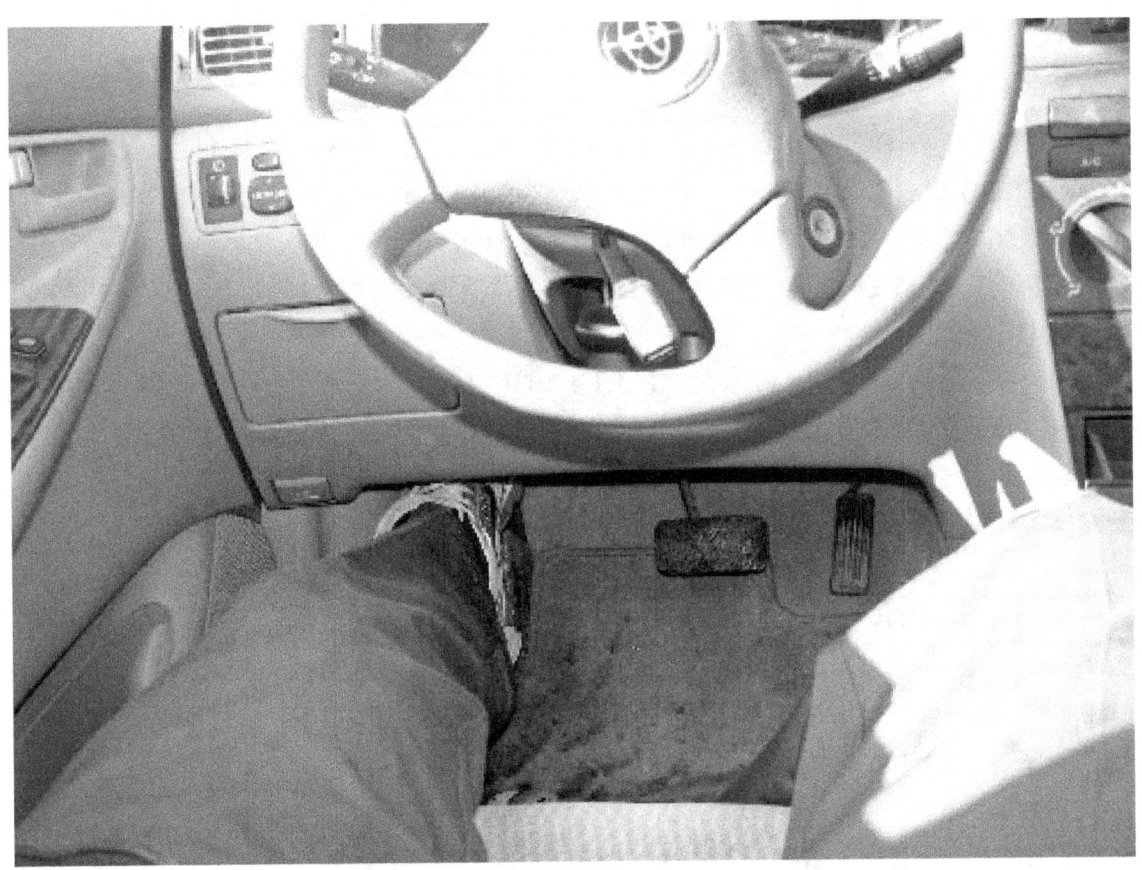

You can do some isometrics for the legs using the resistance of the hard areas above and on either side of your legs, while traffic has come to a standstill or when you have the opportunity to engage your cruise control.

You can do **abduction/adduction** work this way:

Note**

This **refers to moving the legs towards each other or away from each other and hits the inner and outer parts of the legs.**

Push either leg against the hard spot closest to it (I.E., left leg against left console side), Press the leg against the resistance hard, and hold the position for a count of 5-7 seconds or more, repeat with opposite leg on opposite side of console.
Alternatively, push with right leg against LEFT side console to hit the inner thigh area, also pushing hard for a count of at least 5-7 seconds.
Repeat with left leg pushing against right side console.

The other movement you can do similar to the above is to push your legs upward against the dashboard/console area that is directly over the legs.
Use the standard push hard, hold for a count scheme here again.
You can do the legs individually or together.
You can twist the feet in either direction while doing these to hit the legs a little bit differently.

Using the seat

Triceps

You can hit your triceps muscles isometrically simply **by pushing the backs of your arms hard against the seat and holding for a count.**

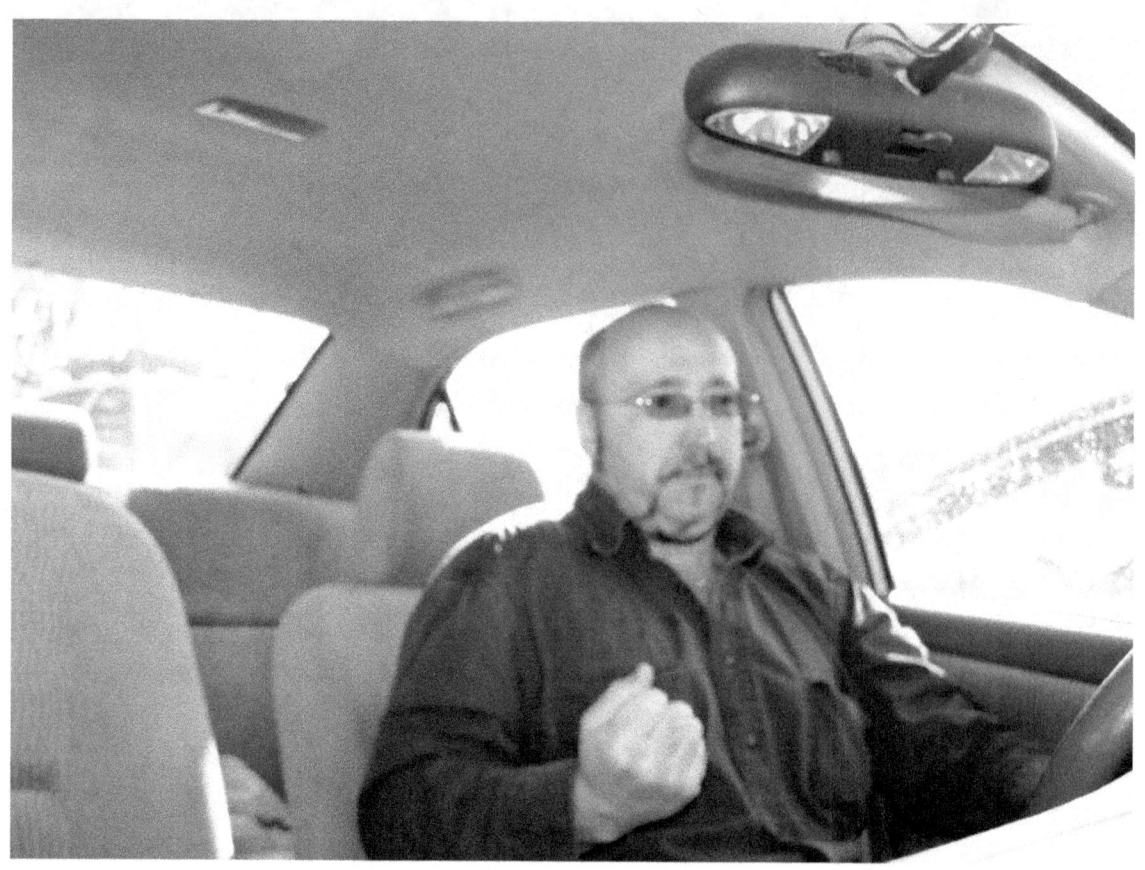

Shoulders

You can reach behind your seat during a traffic stoppage and use your shoulder muscles to push forward against the resistance of the seat.

You can stretch this way by just trying to bring your hands towards each other as far as possible behind your seat, with or without adding in the resistance/holding factor. *You will hit the shoulders a little differently depending on how high or low you grab behind the seat.*

You could grab the underside of your seat and try to "*pull*" it upwards *with your shoulder strength*, also.

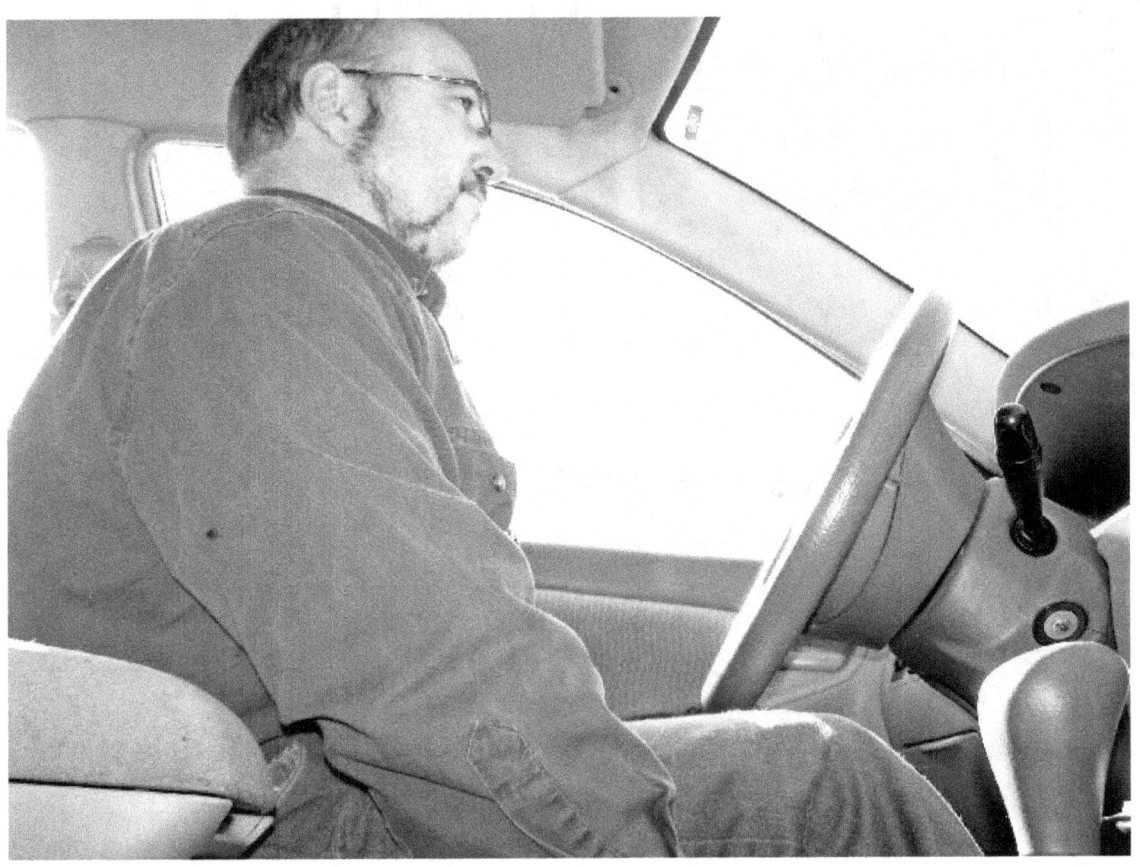

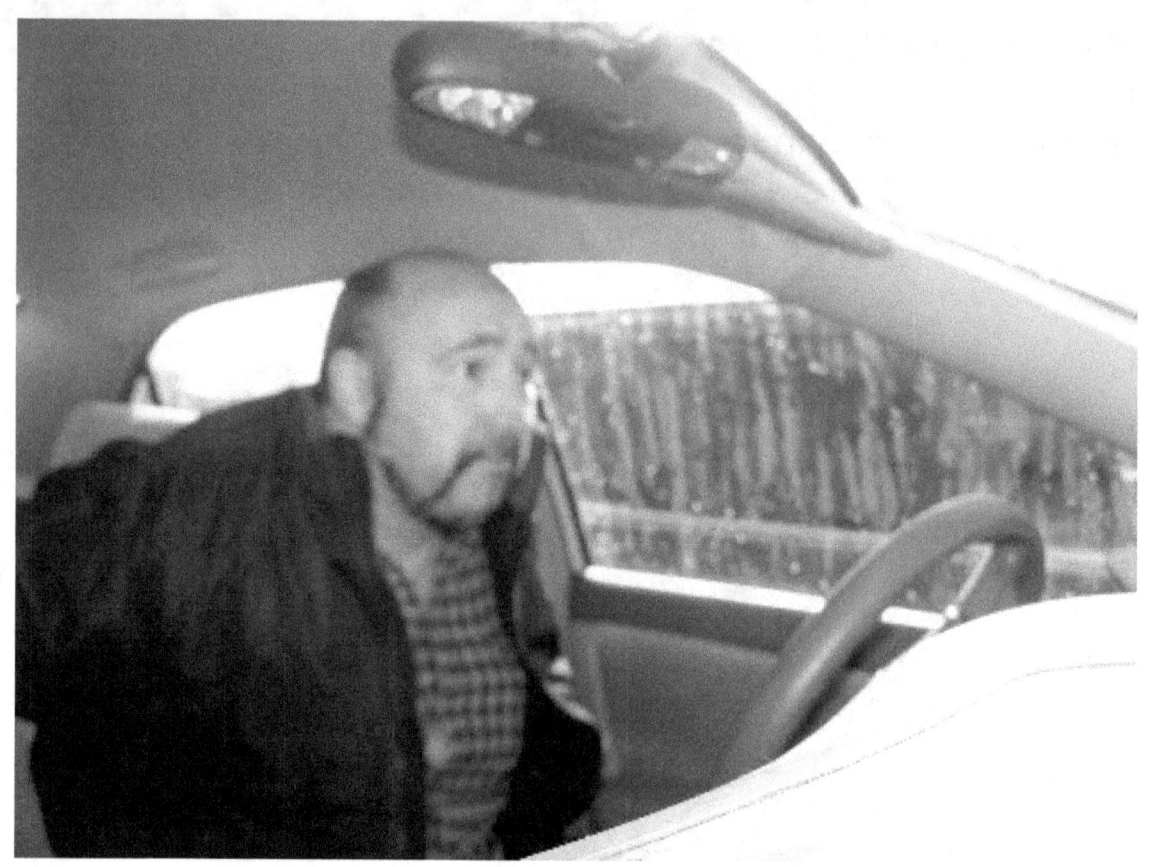

Stretch and/or flex the shoulders while reaching around seat

Biceps

You could also grab under the seat and use your Biceps strength to **pull up on the seat**, using a little bit more of an angle than you used for the shoulder strengthening version, or;

Triceps

Use your triceps muscles to push in against your seat sides, gripping the seat from underneath.

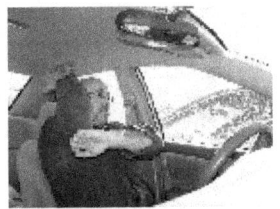

Alternatively,
Use right hand to provide resistance to Triceps pushing downward

Neck

Use your hand as resistance to push your neck against

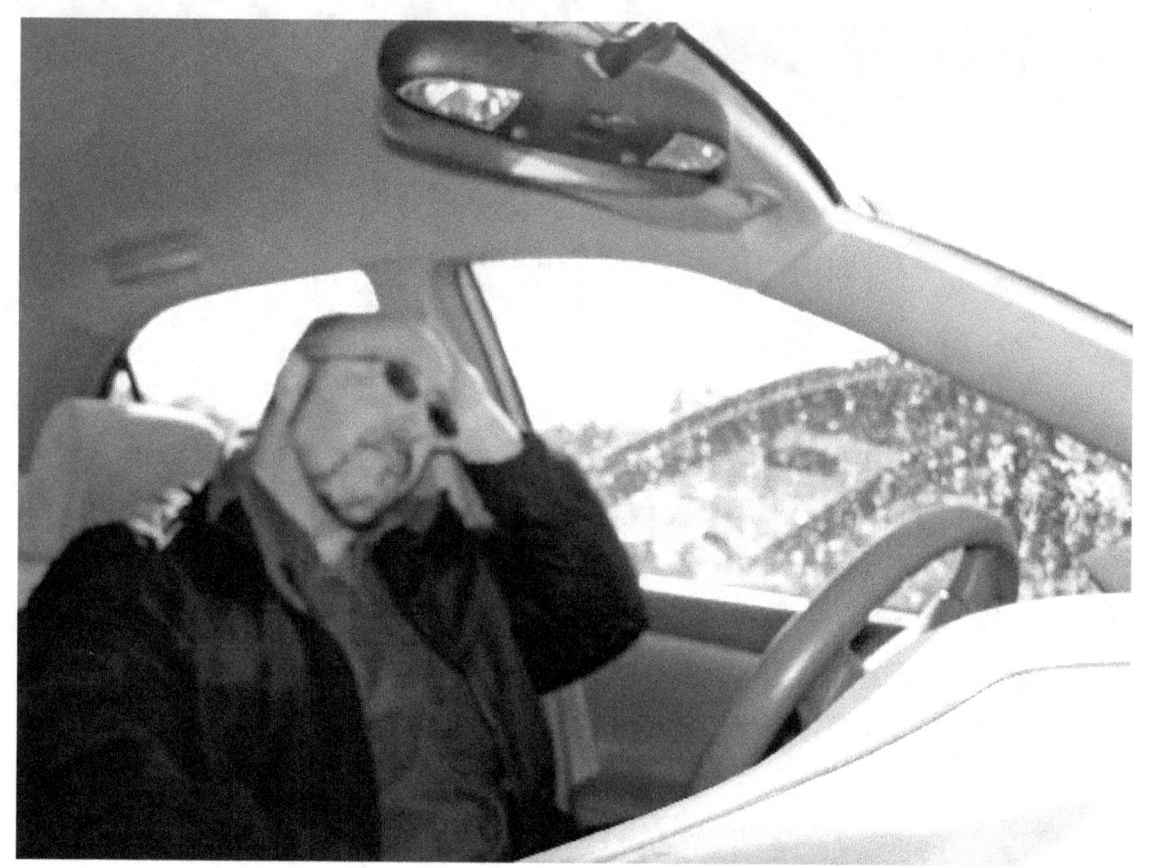

Pushing to left

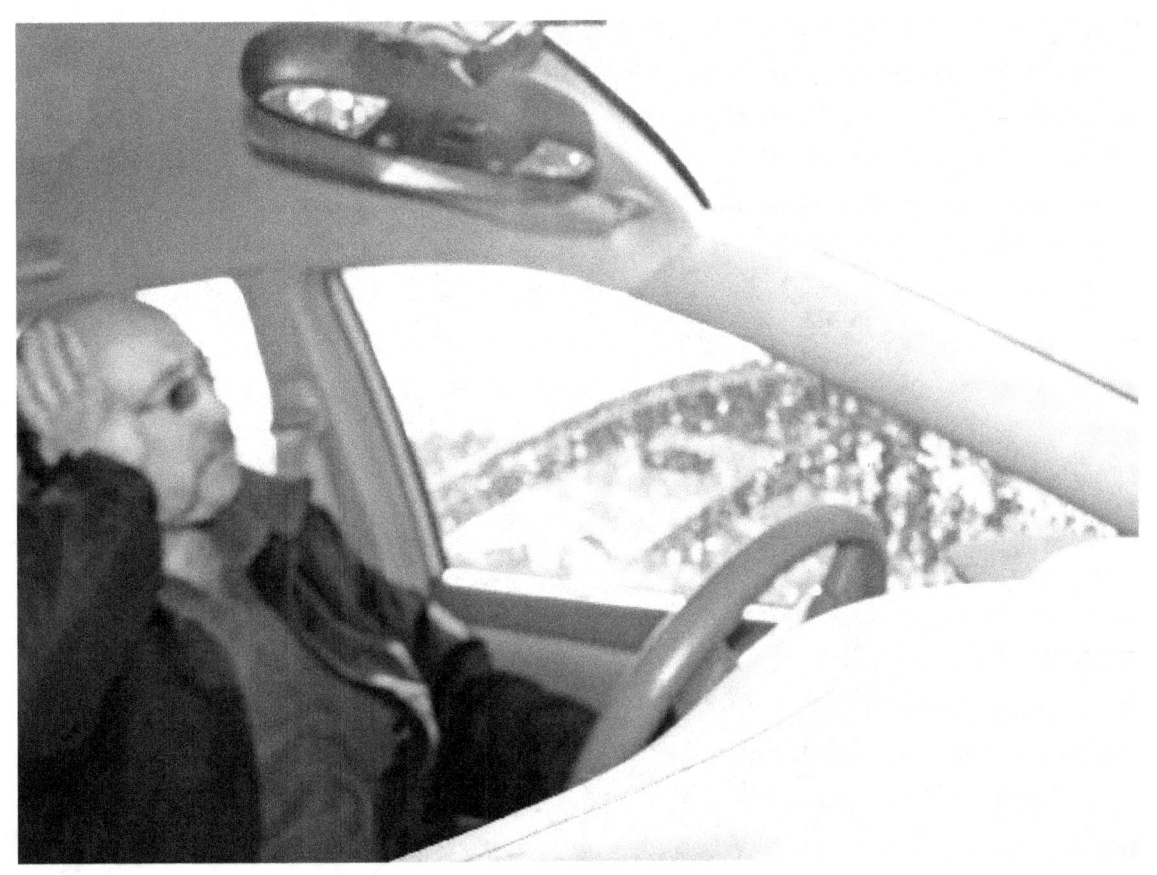

Pushing to right

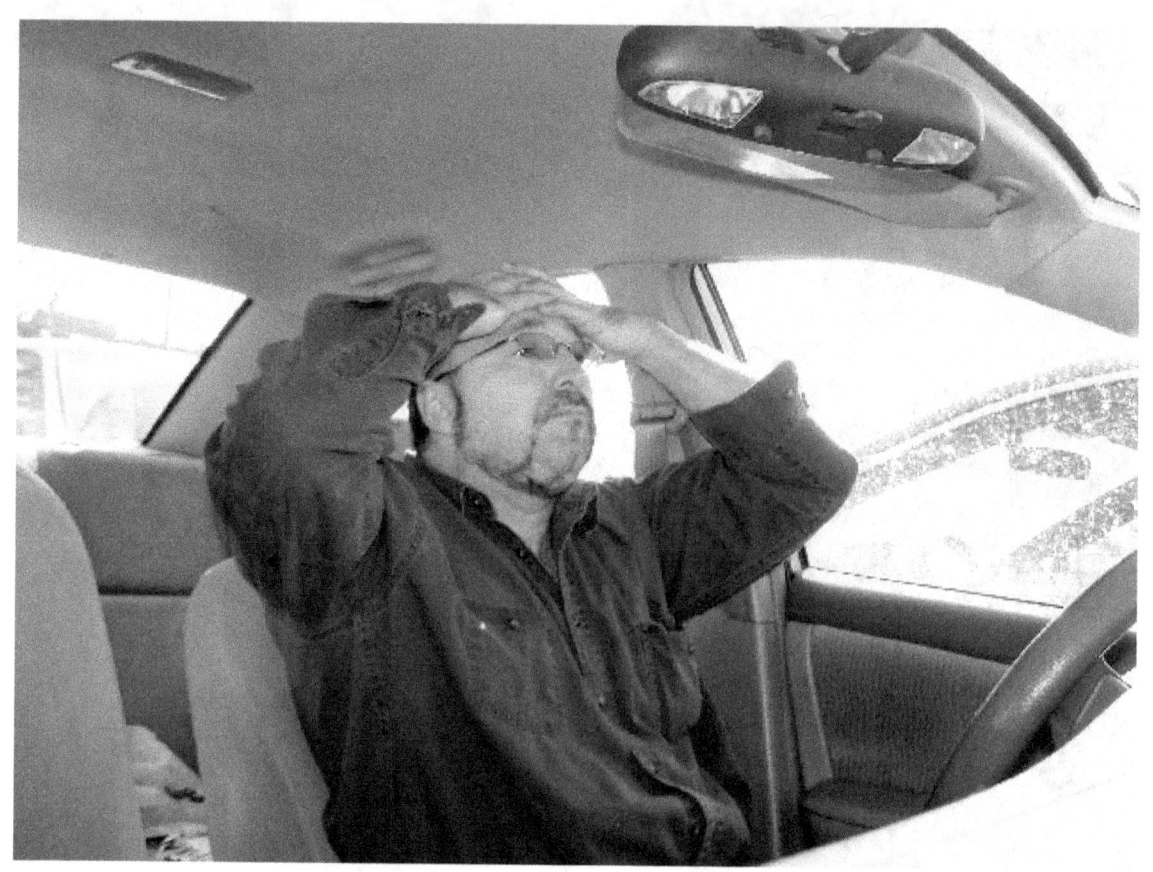

Pushing neck forward against hands

In the next photo, you see the hand putting resistance against the left leg.
The leg is pushing inward against the resistance.

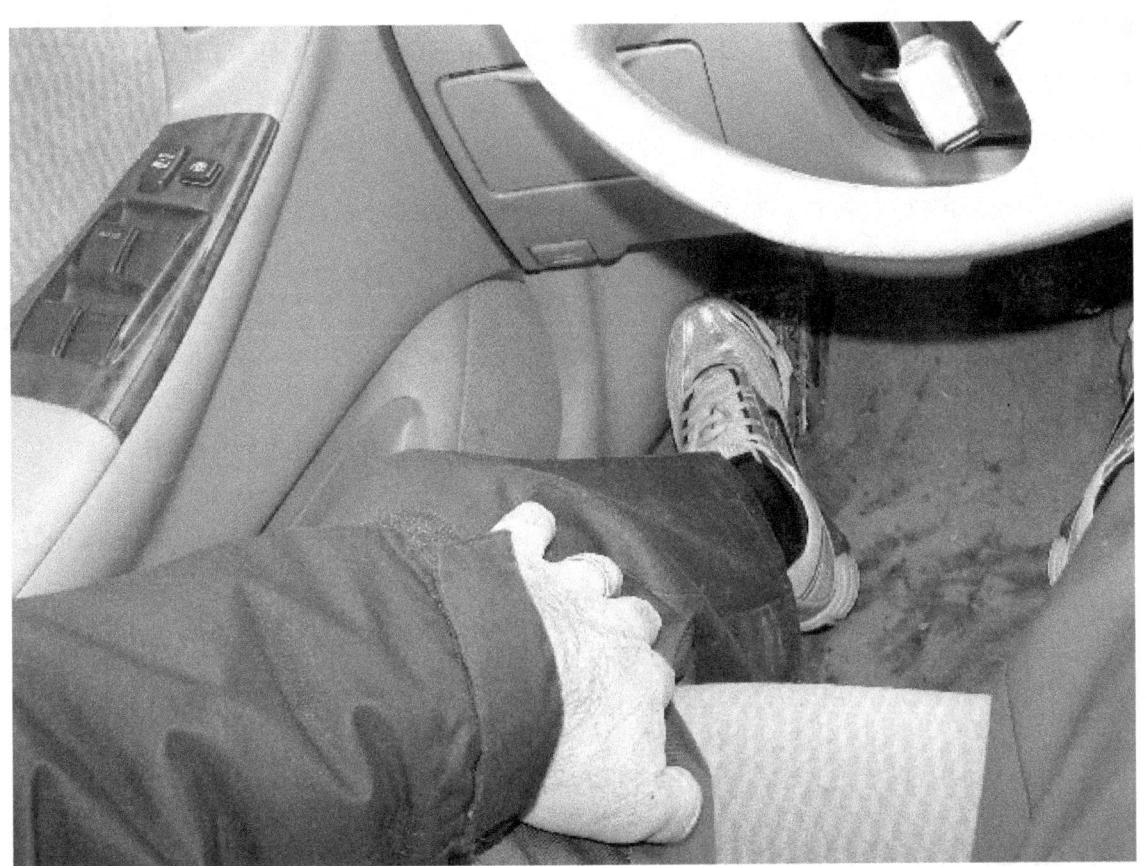

Other resistance types

Place a bag or stack of magazines on your lap to perform heel raises. Lift heels, hold for 8-10 seconds. Relax and then repeat.
Again, you can do this at traffic stops

- **Leg lifts**

- Place an object on the car floor and try lifting it up with your toes.

- It also occurred to me that you could put some **ankle weights on for your commute, and do the leg lifts as the opportunity arises.**

- You could also perform "scissors" with or without ankle weights in situations where your legs are both free, or even a bicycling type of movement, again, with or without the weights. (this will require a larger under dash area)

- If you can manage to perform higher, faster reps with either of the above movements, it could even be considered as a **mild aerobic workout**!

-

Flex tube ideas

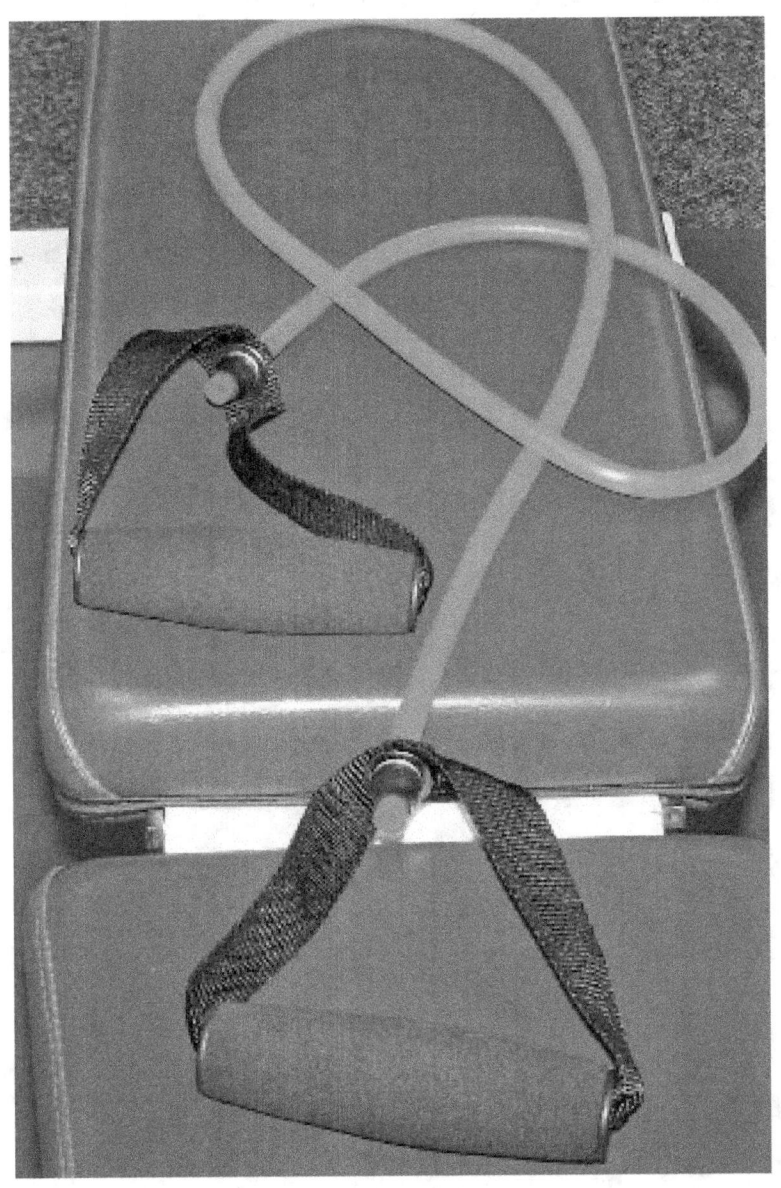

You have probably seen the ***elastic tubing with handles*** at both ends for exercising with.
These are relatively inexpensive and come in various thicknesses which make for varying levels of difficulty.

You can find a way to attach one to your seat, maybe using one of those bags that hang off of the headrest.
You could put some holes on either side of the bag; thread the tube through the holes and so that the handles can be grabbed on either side of your seat.
Put your seat way back and grab the tubing handles and perform chest presses.

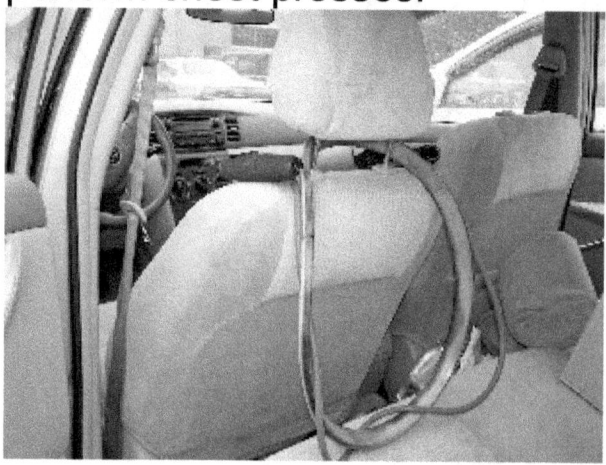

I simply used an old rubber gasket hung off my headrest, with a flex tube threaded through it.
You can place the tube handles on either side of the seat, for easy access at any time.
Make sure both ends are evenly spaced from their anchor point in the middle.

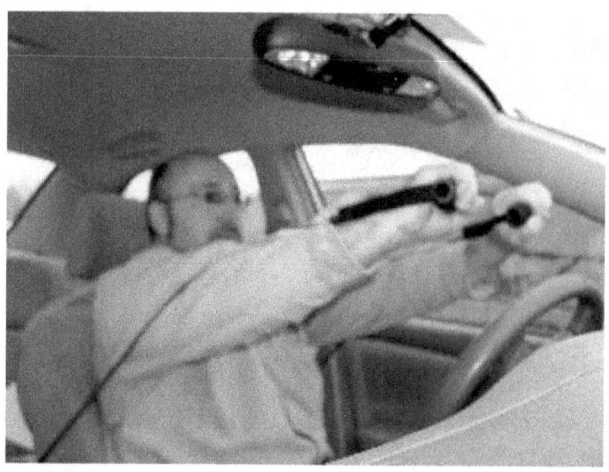

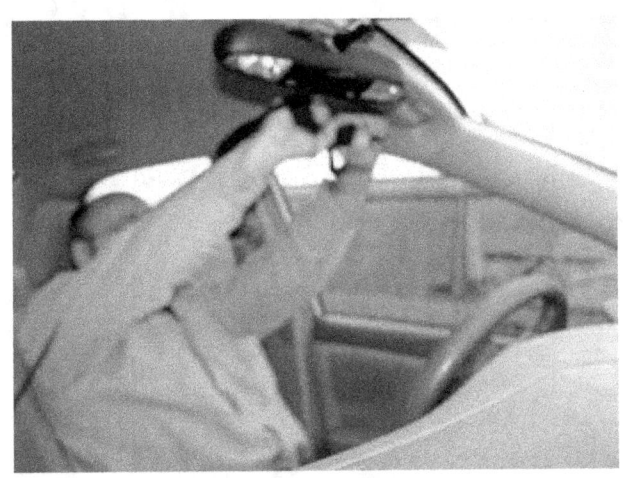

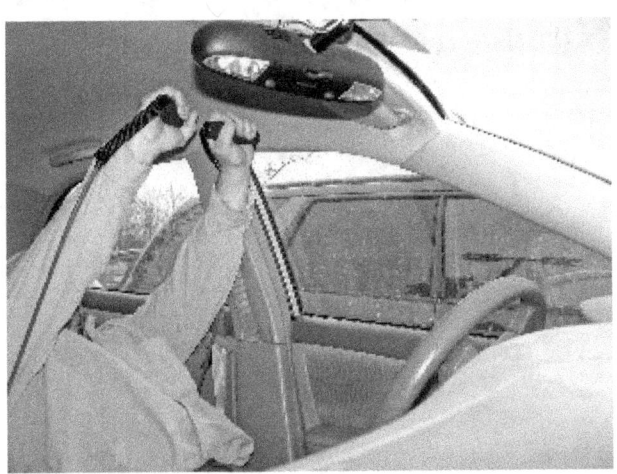

You can bring the handles straight forward, or use an upward angle to hit the upper pecs and deltoids more. Of course, you can only do this during traffic stops!
You could also **run a tube underneath the seat and use it to do bicep curls during stoppages.**

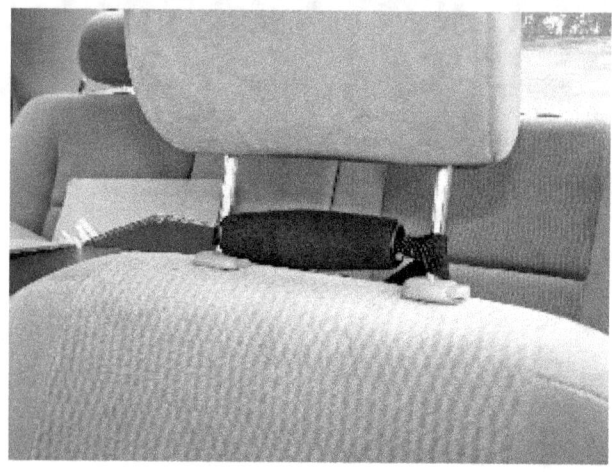

Start by attaching one handle to the headrest as shown.

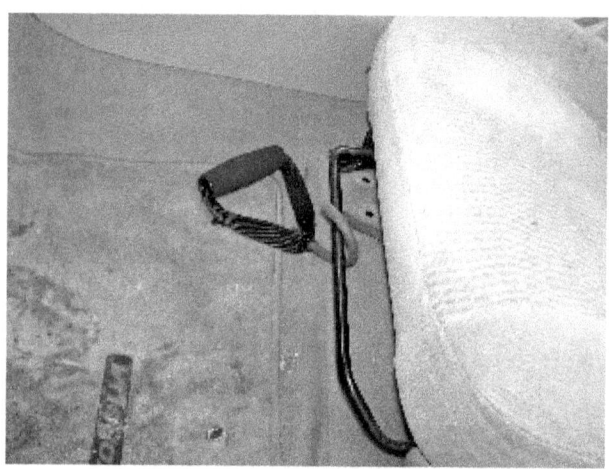

Next, thread tube underneath seat, and you can wrap around seat moving mechanism just to keep in place.

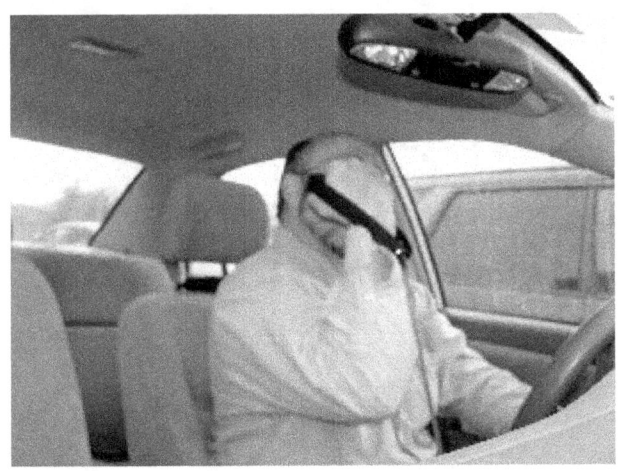

The tube is now available for doing "**curls**" with either arm, or press upwards for shoulder work, as you get the opportunity.

One more idea is to step on the tube and do "**rowing motions**", with the seat tilted way back during a traffic stop. You can simply step on the middle of the tube and pullit up and back with both hands.

"Carobics"

I mentioned in the section above that you could do Scissors or bicycle movements for fast enough and long enough to provide an aerobic workout of sorts.

You could also do high speed, multi-repetition boxing type moves to get some upper body cardio work in.
Put ankle weights above the wrists for an added challenge here, or hold some hand weights like those used when jogging!

"Caristhenics"

During long traffic stops, you can tilt the seat way back; **hook your feet up under the dash/console if that's possible, and perform crunches or sit-ups from this position.**

If you have your ankle weights on, you can simply hold your legs out straight while reclining in your tilted back seat to blast the abdominal section.
Hold the position for as long as you can stand!

You can do the sit-ups like those in the first "**Caristhenics**" exercise mentioned, but this time touch or at least reach for the roof when you come up.
Add a body twist to this move, alternatively, to hit the oblique muscles on the sides.
Twist in opposite directions on each "**rep**".

You could also just keep a stationary upper body position while twisting as far from side to side as possible to hit the same muscles.

Flexing with no external resistance

"Glute squeeze"

Keep your Rear end from getting numb by **squeezing your gluteus muscles**, hold for a count of 10, and then relax. . You can do this one "**cheek**" at a time, or use both simultaneously. Try a little of each method.

"Grab a ticket"

Imagine that you have a winning lottery ticket. **Grasp it and hold it tightly between your cheeks (your Butt cheeks, that is)** count to 10.

Doing this exercise **helps prevent the numbness** in the large gluteus muscles in your posterior that can result from prolonged sitting.

It may also be a good idea to remove wallets from the back pockets since sitting on them can add to the numbness and increase the risk of painful sciatica.

Toe raises

Toe raises will help work the muscles on the front of your shins. Lift toes, hold 10 seconds, relax and repeat.

•

Static abdominal raise

Try tilting your seat back a little farther than the position in which you normally sit, and hold yourself in the

position as if you were still sitting with the seat in your old position
(seat @ 30 degrees, body @20 degrees, or something similar).

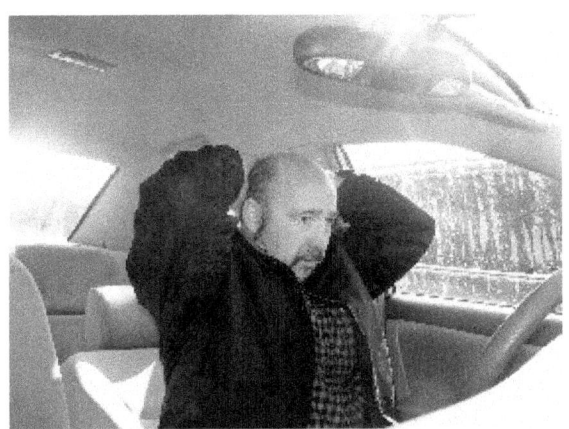

Isolated flexes

The beauty of these exercises is that ***they can target any muscle of the body and require no real movement.***
This makes them ***ideal for doing while driving.***
We really need to learn to flex individual muscle groups in isolation so that we can train different sections on different days when we need to.

Upper Back

Lat flare/contract

The "*lats*" are the **Latissimus Dorsi** muscles.
They are the **wing like muscles** of the upper back that create width.
Flare the lats out as wide as you can while also flexing/contracting them as hard as possible and holding that position for 5-7 seconds.
You should do both sides at the same time on this one, although you could do each side individually.

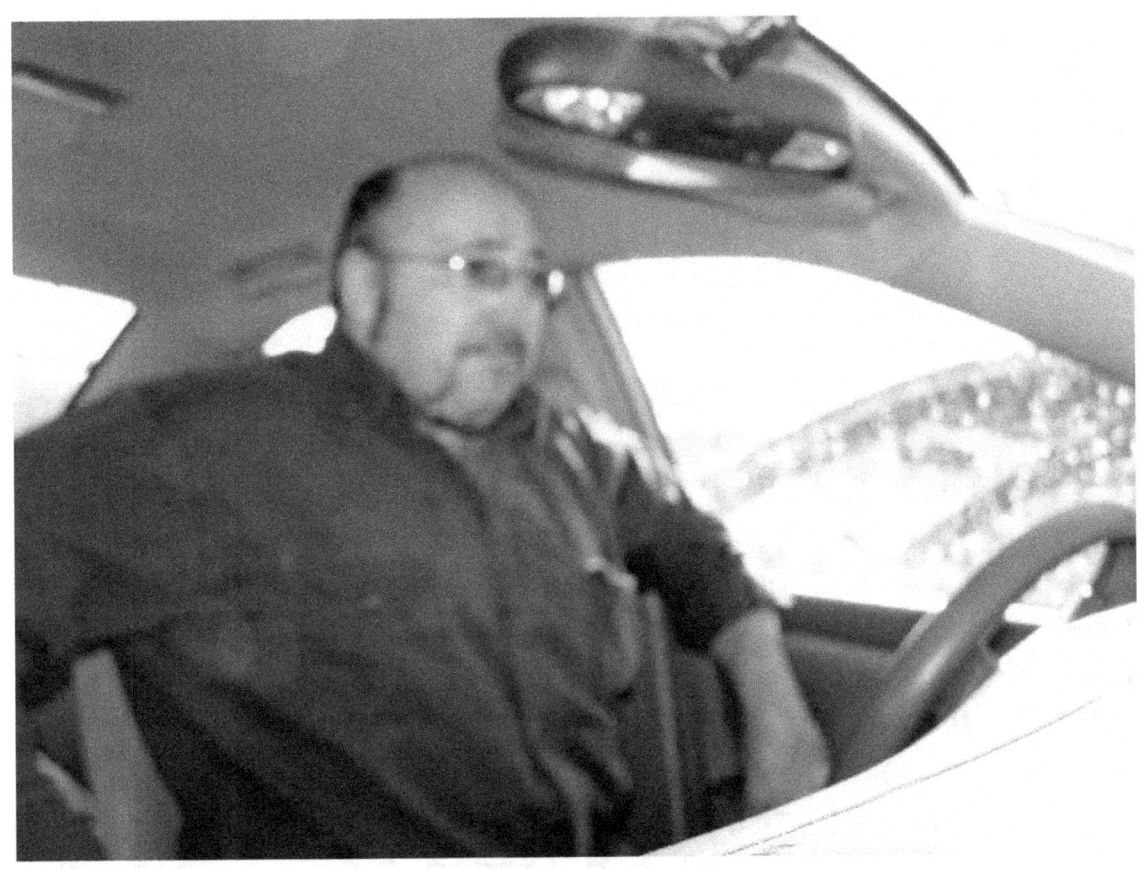

Now try to concentrate on the middle back and flex/contract that area.

Try and "**push**" your backs muscles in towards your stomach, and towards each other, and hold the position again for 5-7 seconds once more here.
To finish the upper back, **shrug the shoulders up as high as possible while flexing/contracting the trapezius muscles (the muscles between your shoulders and your neck**)
Hold as in the last 2 moves.

Biceps

Earlier in the book, I mentioned the old "*make a muscle*" idea relating to flexing and contracting the biceps muscles. It helps in contracting the biceps to **make a fist**, and then to twist the wrist inward somewhat. Ideally, you want the elbow joint "*closed*" as if you had just picked a weight up starting from the arm extended position.

As always, hold the contracted position for 5-7 seconds. *You can also flex the biceps hard with arm in various stages of flexion, like fully extended, halfway closed or anywhere in between.*

One of the old time fitness gurus, **Joe Bonom**o used a technique he called "*Vibro-power*" in which you would hold a flexed position so forcefully and for so long that the flexed part would start to vibrate.

The arm is a good place to start when first trying this method.

Simply "*point*" your finger at something straight ahead, *flexing your whole arm while pointing.*

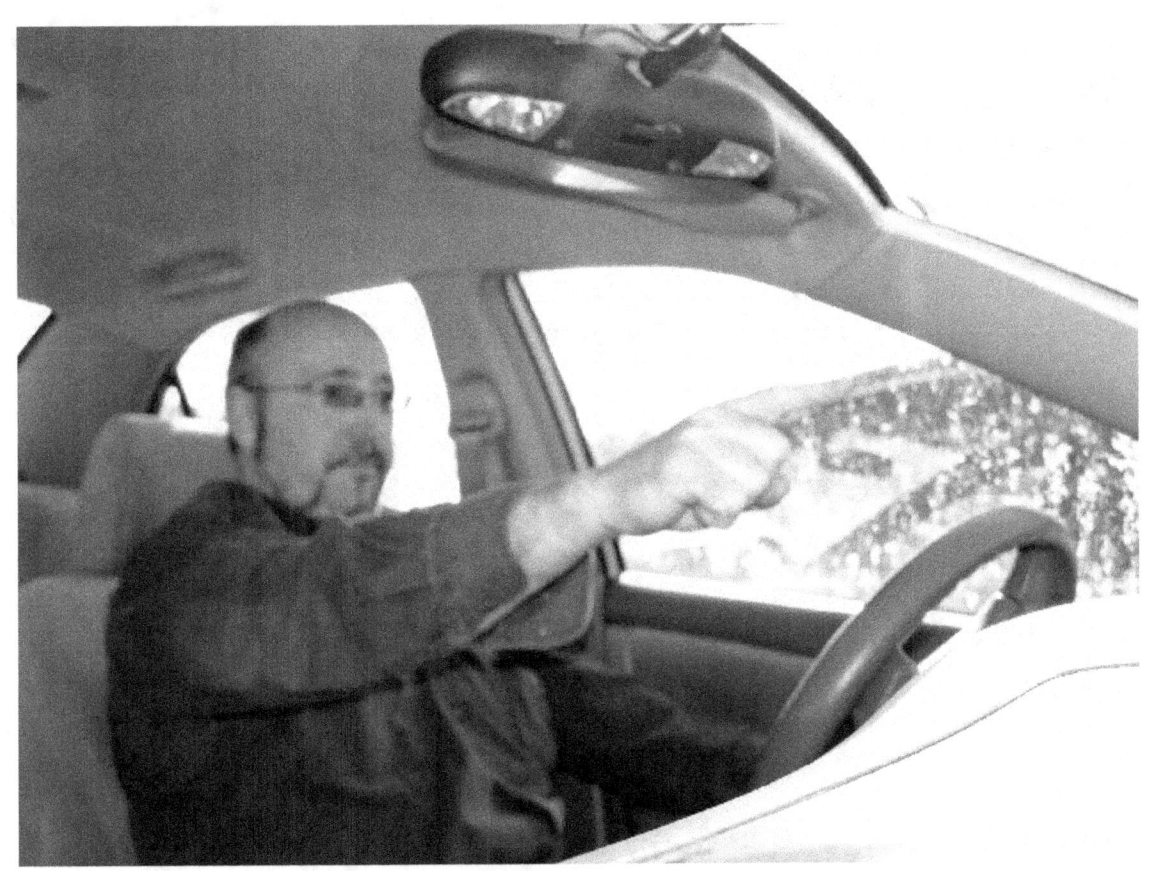

Try to keep ***increasing the flex tension as you continue to hold the position, and continue increasing the tension until the entire arm begins to shake or vibrate***.
Once the vibration level has been reached, it will be tough to continue much longer without the muscle cramping up eventually.
We do not want to take it quite to that point.
Once you learn this technique, you can use it to make any of the flexing positions that much more intense.

Once you start to get the hang of this *isolated flexing* idea, You can isolate any muscle group or area you want to work on at any given time.

You can isolate just your shoulders, your abs, your butt muscles or "Glutes", your upper back as we started with above, your upper thighs, your calves, etc.

Abs

The abdominal area is composed of a number of different muscle structures and is therefore not quite as straight-forward in using the isolation flexing methods.

The simplest movement is simply to "*suck in the gut*" as if we were at the beach, trying to make an impression. (Don't act like you don't know what I'm talking about, please)

You can just suck in the gut and hold it in tightly for several minutes or more. Use your clock, and start the contraction just as the minute changes.

A *variation* I have been doing is to *suck the stomach in and to one side at the same time, and then push it out towards the middle, followed by pulling in towards the opposite side.*

I continue this for an entire minute or more, or for a certain number of repetitions to each side.

Pull the stomach muscles *up and in tightly* to each side on each contraction.

I can tell you if you really concentrate on these and continue the contractions for a full 2 minutes or more, you will really feel as if you had just done a bunch of sit-ups.

When I do the simpler "gut suck-ins", I try to pull the stomach **up towards the chest and back towards the spine at the same time.**
It helps me to try and start with a "mild" contraction and to then gradually build the intensity of the contraction, much like the previously mentioned "**Vibro-Power**" idea, but not taking it to the point of shaking or vibrating at the final stages.

The Role of the Mind

The role of the mind is **extremely important in getting the most benefit from these exercises.**
It absolutely can not be over emphasized!
The level to which you are able to flex/contract any muscle without actually pushing a weight or pulling against some "real" resistance will be **utterly dependant on your ability to focus and concentrate on doing it**.
Like anything else, practice makes perfect in this exercise mode.
Keep working at it and you will get better and better at it.

Legs

Flexing the upper legs or the lower legs is reasonably straight-forward, with the exception that you may want to try and isolate the front of the legs from the back.
I strongly encourage learning to do it both ways; that is; to try flexing the entire upper leg area including the hamstrings and the quadriceps first, and then try and isolate the front thigh (quadriceps) muscle from the hamstring muscles or back of the leg.

You can isolate the front and back of the lower legs very easily.
Raising the heel and flexing will **emphasize the back or calves, while raising the toes and flexing will work the Soleus,** at the front of the lower leg.

We talked about flexing the "**glutes**" or butt muscles earlier, so we'll leave that alone at this point.

Pecs

The pectoral muscles of the chest, known as the "**pecs**", are one of the favorite muscle groups of bodybuilders everywhere.

They are not too difficult to isolate and flex, following the same flex and hold for a 5-7 count as we did in the previous exercises.

Triceps

Concentrate on just the back of the arms and flex hard and hold in the prescribed fashion. The **Triceps are the muscles that are in the back of the arms.**
The Triceps typically work together with the pectoral muscles in what we refer to as the "**pushing**" movements.

Forearms

The forearms can be done simultaneously with the biceps when performing the "**pointing**" exercise we discussed previously.
They can also be done in the more "isolated" fashion.

Keep in mind that the wrists, hands and forearms are all tied together, and that turning the wrists in different positions, squeezing the hands in different ways, etc., will make subtle changes in the way the forearm muscles contract while flexing.

Lower back

This is the one primary area we have not already discussed, but it certainly bears talking about.

This is an area that can be difficult to flex without some movement being added.

I suggest moving the whole lower body forward a bit, while thrusting (slowly moving back) the upper body back into the top of the seat as a starting point for lower back flexion.

Once you have reached that position, it is easier to focus on flexing the lower back in an isolated fashion.

The further down and back the upper back is placed, the more stretch is put on the lower back.

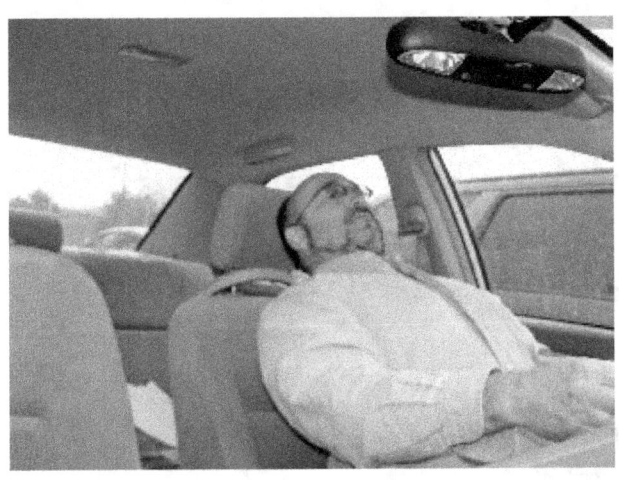

Stretching/flexing the lower back

That pretty much covers the pure *isolation flexing movements.*

KSHD

Now, we can move on, into the **Kin Shi Hai Do** movements.
As we already talked about, this concept refers to the idea of
"*virtual*" weightlifting.
You can simply "*visualize*" lifting a barbell or dumbbell,
pulling down a bar that is connected to a stack of weights,
etc.

As opposed to the isolated flexing positions we went through in the last section, this involves **going through the entire range of motion** of specific typical weight training or other types of exercises without the "normal" resistance in a physical sense.

Again, the **mind plays a crucial role in the effectiveness of this method.**

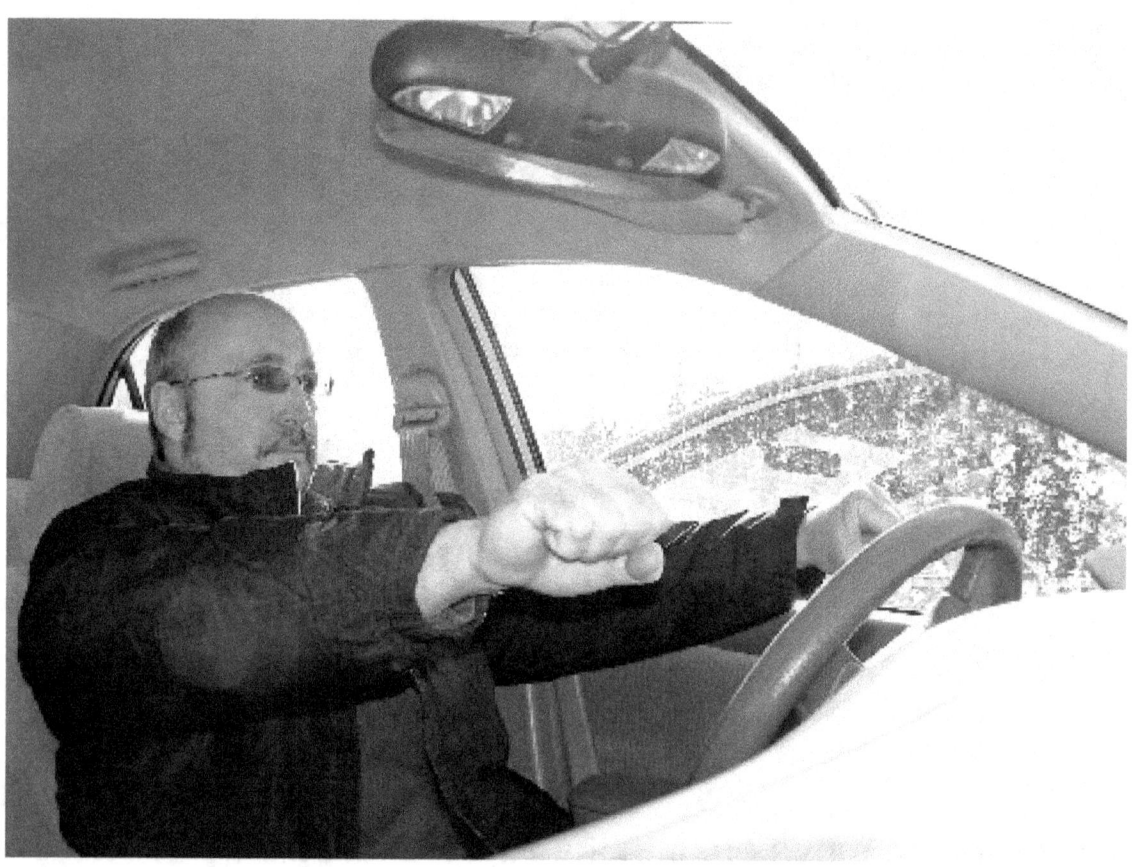

KSHD Simulated Bench Press shown at lockout position

You can "*virtually*" perform any typical exercise that you might wish to, simply by imagining that you are actually curling a dumbbell, pressing a barbell, or whatever.
With a good imagination, you can imagine yourself doing any exercise possible.
You can even "invent" your own machine or apparatus in your mind, which **enables you to perform any exercise you can think of!**

You can do "*virtual*" bench presses, military presses, curls, whatever comes to your mind.

You can perform the exercises with several variations.
You can opt to concentrate only on the "*positive*" part of a movement (*concentric phase*), only on the relaxing part where the muscle *returns to its original position (eccentric phase), or use both phases.*

At this point, we should discuss concentric and eccentric contractions in a little more in-depth fashion.

When you perform a standard bicep curl, "*pulling*" a weight up to the point where your arm is fully contracted, elbow closed, you have just completed the "*concentric*" phase.
When you let the weight return back to its original position, with arm fully extended, you have just completed the "*eccentric phase*".
In typical weight training exercises, the concentric phase is usually emphasized.
Putting the concentration on the eccentric phase can be extremely demanding.
If one would load a bar to a weight somewhat beyond what they could bench press (for example), and have a couple of spotters standing by, they could "fight" the descent of the loaded bar to the starting point.

I have tried this method and believe me; you will get very sore afterwards!

The point I am trying to make is that you can concentrate on the concentric, the eccentric or both phases of any exercise when doing "*virtual resistance*" training.

You can **keep the muscles tensed throughout any particular movement, just keep tensed for either the concentric or eccentric phase, or just contract hard at any specific point of the full range of motion of the exercise.**

Using more conventional training equipment in your car

There are some smaller, unobtrusive pieces of equipment that can be used in a conventional, if somewhat limited fashion, in your car.
Various **gripping devices** using springs, thick rubber balls, etc., come to mind as being easy to use with one hand while driving with the other.
You can use **flex-tubes** as described already earlier, during traffic stops.
You could even use a **bullworker** or similar type of "**live isometric**" device during traffic stops.

Spring Gripper (modified)

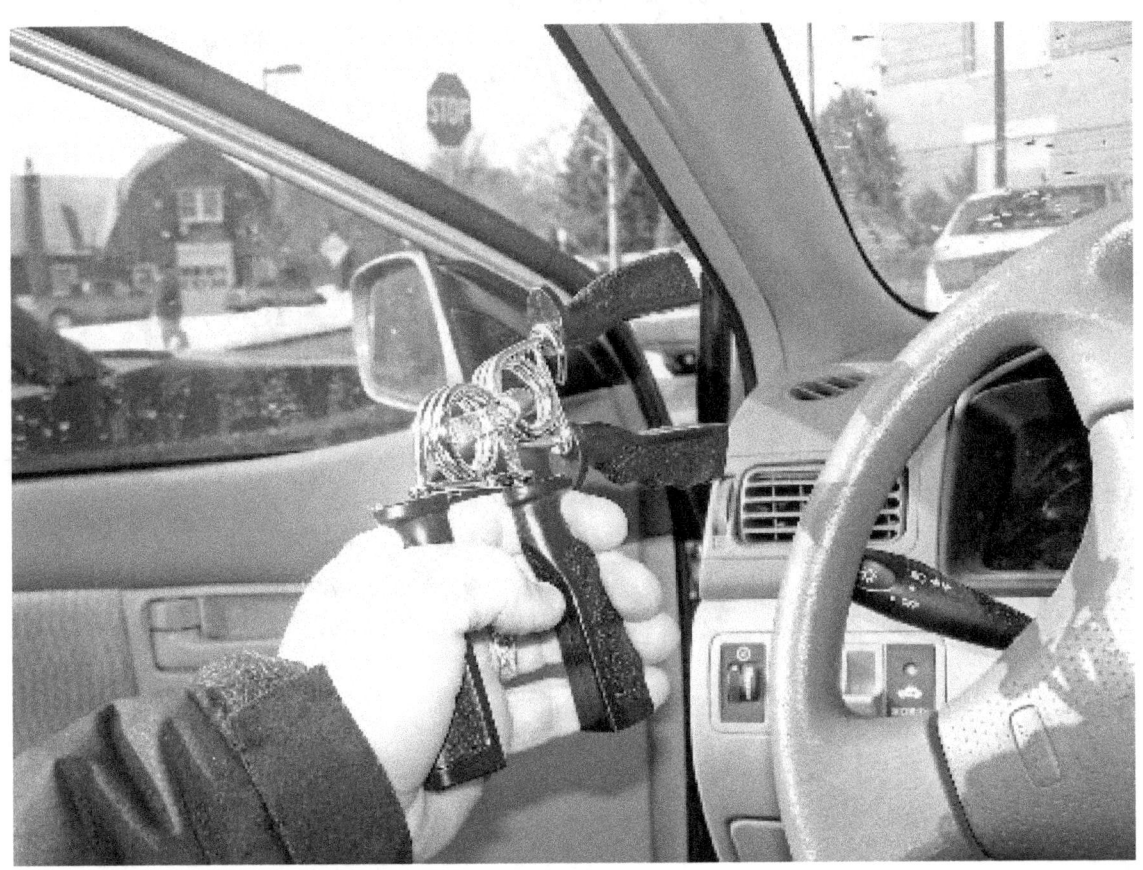

Bullworker shown on photo

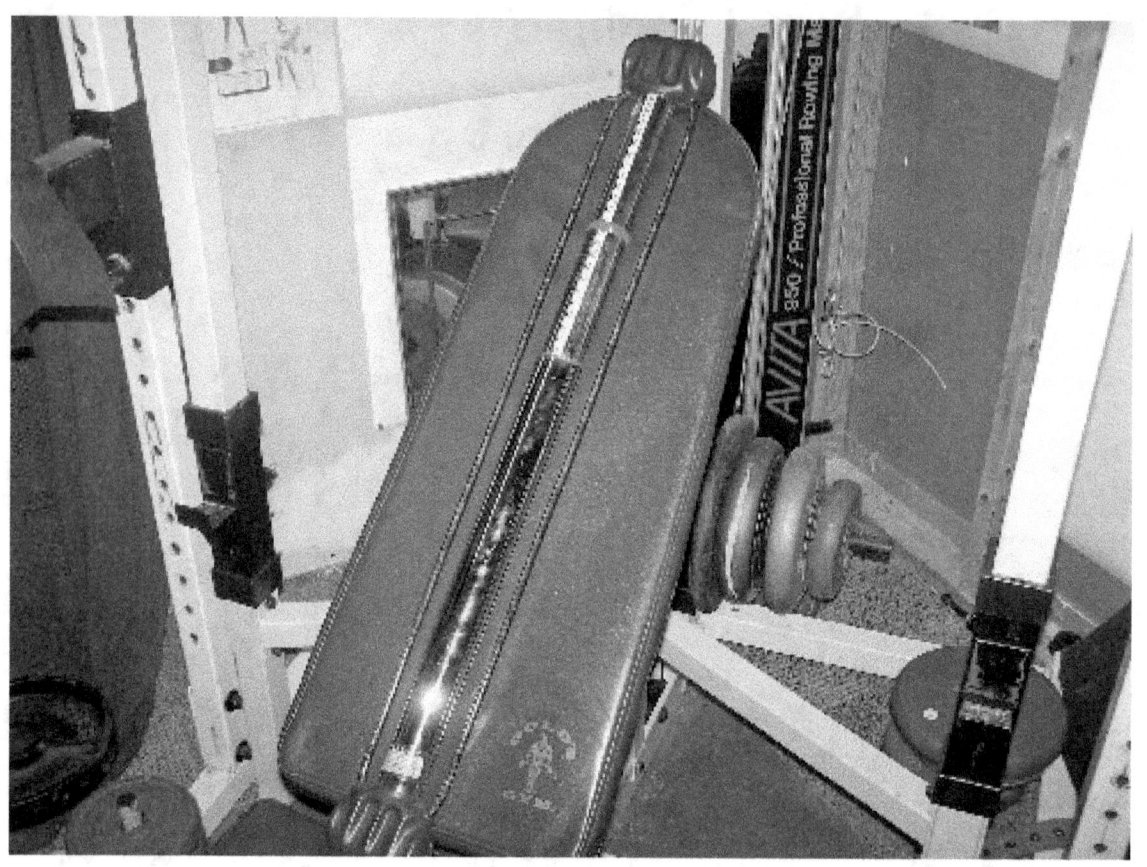

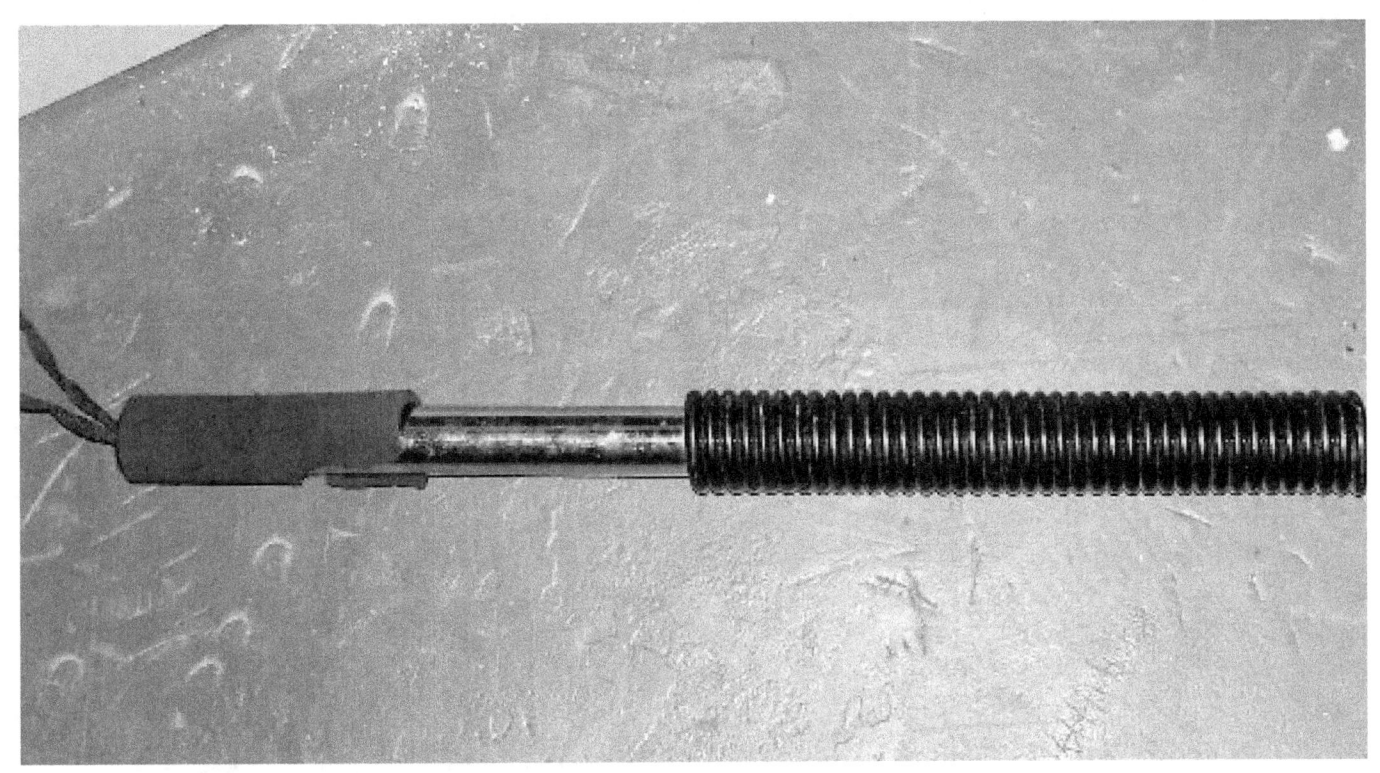

Spring bar

Again, putting some **ankle weights** on before your commute starts will enable you to do **weighted leg lifts** and such during stoppages.

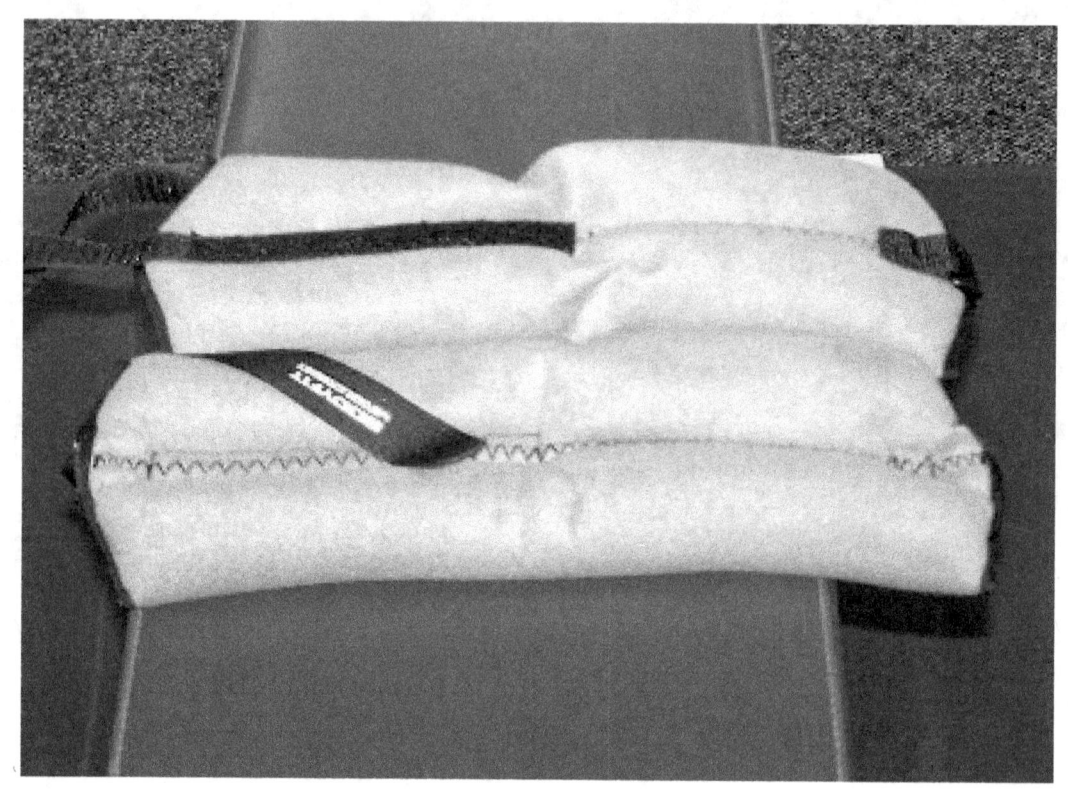

Ankle weights

Putting it all together

You can easily switch back and forth between isolation flexes, isometrics, KSHD and stretching movements in every possible combination imaginable.

And then, of course there are the **deep breathing** methods we also talked about earlier.
I encourage practicing the **deep breathing techniques in between doing the other exercises.**

I have endeavored to give you a full "**tool box**" from which to draw from in this book.
As I said from the start, however, getting all of the exercise you need in your car will be difficult at best.

There are numerous relatively easy ways to incorporate other forms of exercise into your everyday routine.

One of the most obvious things that come to mind is that when you reach your destination after your typical commute, you are going to park somewhere.
Normally, you might choose to park as close as possible to your office, or other workplace.

Instead of parking as close as possible to your destination, try parking at the opposite end of the lot and getting a little walk in.

If this seems too hard at first, compromise and just park a little farther away than normal, and then try and stretch the distance a bit at a time.

When you are at work, *try taking the stairs instead of the elevator when commuting between floors.*

You can really use the stairs to get a killer workout if you have the time and the inclination.

A set of stairs can be a cheap and uncomplicated way to get a workout, and *you can perform a workout in any building that has stairs.*

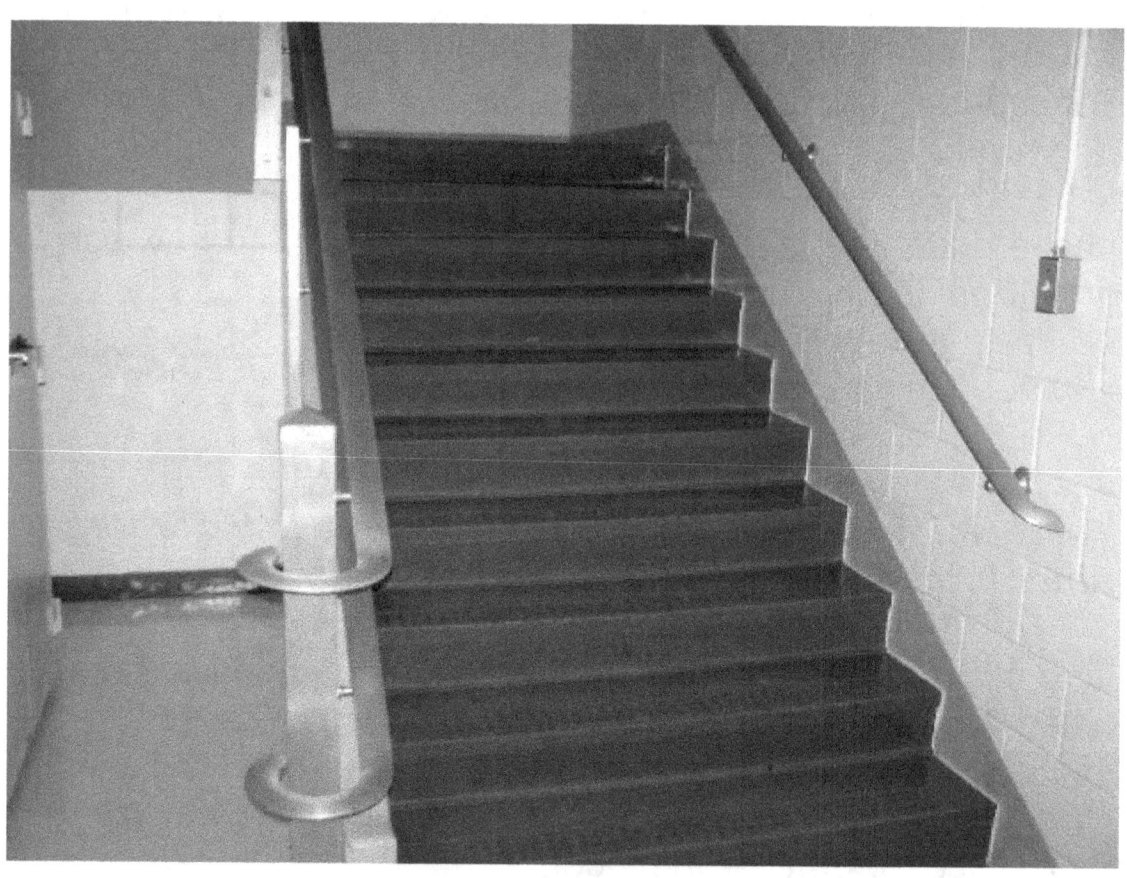

It can be as simple as walking the stairs instead of taking the elevator, or can graduate to running up the steps hard, skipping 2 or 3 steps at a time, bounding from side to side as you run up the steps, and more.

You can also do **step-ups and lunges on the stairs**; add difficulty to walking or running the stairs by **adding ankle weights, holding small weights or adding a weight vest.** (You could just put some weight in a back pack for the frugal version of this)

If your workplace does not have the luxury of a gym on site, you can still **find ways to get a workout in**. Take a **jump rope** along and maybe a **set of flex tubes** also, and find a spot outside or a vacant room to get a quick workout in during coffee breaks or your lunch hour.

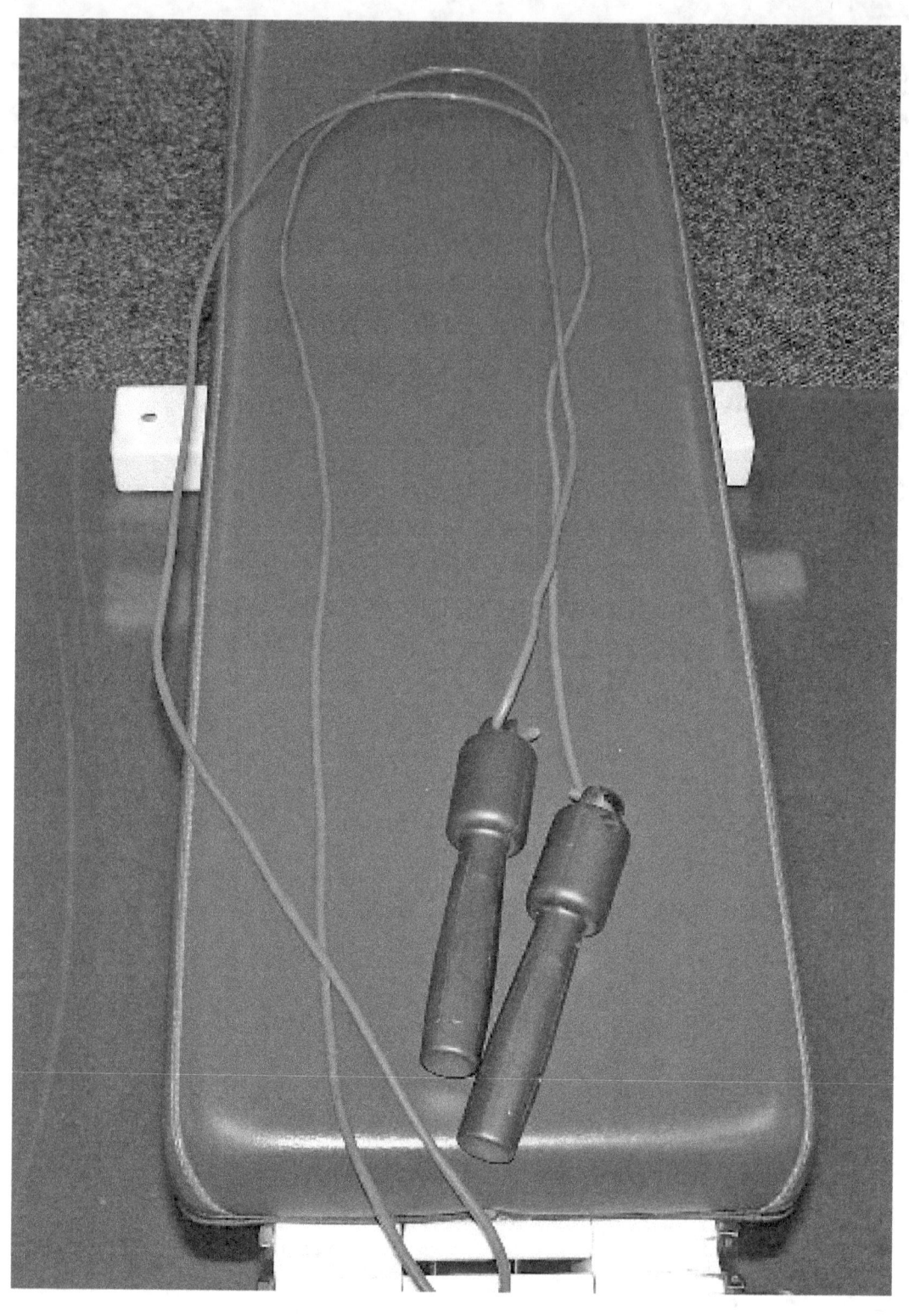

Jump Rope

Of course, you can do most or all of the exercises we've discussed doing on your commute, **at your desk.**

From a minimalist standpoint, **you should at least add some form of cardio training to your car workouts for a better rounded fitness routine.**

The little pedometers that you put on your belt or hip somewhere can be nice little **motivational tools**, as well as helping you to measure your progress.

Try to **add steps during your workday**, in the ways I already mentioned. This will burn calories and "**rev up**" your metabolism a notch.

If you have been relatively sedentary, this is a good place to start, and will not over-tax your heart and lungs too much.

This does not require a gym membership, a big outlay financially, or much of a time commitment, so there's little excuse not to do it if you truly want to improve your physical conditioning.

Also keep in mind that you can do all of the car exercises that we have suggested **in your living room, while watching T.V., etc.**

Another concept is to consider normal "**chores**" like shoveling snow, mowing the lawn, gardening, etc as a workout.

This helps to put a more positive perspective on things, I think.

Try getting up to change the channel on the T.V. instead of using the remote all the time.

Park, get out of your car and walk into the fast food restaurant (if you are forced to make that choice), instead of going through the drive-through.

By the way, there are some not-so- horrible foods available at fast food restaurants these days, if you look hard enough.

For more tips, videos, personal training services, links and much more, please consider stopping by my website at

http://Christianiron.com